Intelligent Kindness

Reforming the Culture of Healthcare

D0791793

John Ballatt and Penelope Campling

RCPsych Publications

Photograph of healthcare worker p. 173: the publishers have been unable to determine copyright in this image.

RCPsych Publications is an imprint of the Royal College of Psychiatrists,
17 Belgrave Square, London SW1X 8PG
http://www.rcpsych.ac.uk

British Library Cataloguing-in-Publication Data.
A catalogue record for this book is available from the British Library.

ISBN 978-1-908020-04-8

Distributed in North America by Publishers Storage and Shipping Company.

Printed in the UK by Bell & Bain Limited, Glasgow.

Contents

Foreword by Tim Dartington   iv

Acknowledgements   viii

Introduction   1

Part I: Healthy kindness

1 Rescuing kindness   9

2 A politics of kindness   18

3 Building the case for kindness   33

Part II: The struggle with kindness

4 Managing feelings of love and hate   51

5 The emotional life of teams   68

6 Cooperation and fragmentation   84

7 On the edges of kinship   100

8 The end of life   115

Part III: The organisation of kindness

9 Unsettling times   125

10 The pull towards perversion   139

11 Free to serve the public   154

12 Intelligent kindness   175

Index   190

Foreword

Tim Dartington

This is a generous book, as befits its subject. It is generous in at least three ways: it explains important ideas in an open and understandable language; it explores theories that are actually useful in thinking about how we care for others; and it offers some comfort for those who work at a difficult time for public services and those (all of us in the end) who need these services.

It is also a whistleblower of a book. Not that it makes sensational accusations or revelations about the unintended cruelties of our health systems; there has been a succession of surveys, reports and inquiries which have done that for us, if we will only take note. This book does something else: it helps us to listen to what we know – from those reports as well as from our own experience – about the difficulties of responding with ordinary kindness to the distress of others. It helps us to overcome our indifference, to face up to the need to do better according to the demands of our humanity.

Who are 'we'? Clinicians, managers, regulators, policy analysts, leaders and followers in the delivery of services to people, when they are at their most vulnerable, when they are sick, distressed, lacking the capacity to look after themselves in a society that rewards enterprise and opportunity and responds to dependency with fear and anxiety.

It is difficult to talk about kindness, an ordinary quality caught up in the technological claptrap. Not sentimental. Not clever. Not easy to audit. As Michael Morpurgo said in his 2011 Richard Dimbleby lecture on the needs of children, you cannot have a league table of relationships. Being with patients, clients, service users can be very hard work. If we deny that as a fact, we are in trouble, because then we build our defences against the difficulty of the work. We try not to feel the pain of the other or our own pain in responding. We have protocols and procedures, form-filling and training days. But this book poses a question for all of us to answer in our own way: how we do things, our practices and systems, are they helpful or are they hindrances to our capacity to show kindness in our relationships? Arguing that kinship and kindness, properly understood, can themselves shape the quality, effectiveness and efficiency of care, John Ballatt and Penelope Campling undertake a wide-ranging exploration of the conditions that influence the expression of those qualities in individuals, teams and organisations.

The authors know what they are talking about. They dig into their extensive clinical and managerial experience to uncover from below the surface the deeply held concern that what we are doing is actually not good enough. They usefully draw on the Department of Health inquiry (the 'Francis Report') into Mid-Staffordshire NHS Foundation Trust, in which the new medical director was praised for saying 'Our job is to treat patients, that is all there is to it'. They ask 'How have we come to reach such a state of affairs that this simple statement sounds so radical?'

We often want to see the failures of a system as isolated incidents, aberrations in an otherwise well-functioning state of affairs. But there are too many failures for this to be a sustainable argument. The Francis Report is just one in a series that stretches back in the history of health and social welfare and that will undoubtedly continue into the future. In the same few months, we have heard further stories of abuse from the Patients Association and the Parliamentary and Health Service Ombudsman.

Our public services are always being reorganised – new initiatives and reforms overtake each other like waves on the beach. There is no use complaining about this destabilising political leadership – it will always be so. This is the product of a deep anxiety, felt most acutely perhaps by politicians and their economic advisers, that responding to the needs of others will drag us down in a slough of dependency. But human needs do not change in any fundamental way, and those who look to work in the interests of vulnerable people will continue to find ways of overcoming the obstacles put in their way by such anxiety-driven changes. That is the hope as we learn to live with efficiency savings that are neither efficient nor saving.

The book is very easy to read, and at the same time very difficult. What Ballatt and Campling are saying is important, chronically true and acutely relevant at this time. They describe how kind people do unkind things, and how unkind people – the same people – get away with it for so long. They explore the questions 'How do good staff become bad?' and 'How do we prevent that happening?' It is necessary to manage our feelings and to do this we need both protective space and support. So they make the case for staff support groups, in the tradition first of Balint groups for doctors and 'Schwarz rounds', a US initiative. There is, I would add, a lively tradition of reflective and reflexive work by front-line staff in the work discussion groups developed by the Tavistock Clinic in London. The authors foreground human qualities rather than competencies in the delivery of care.

The middle section develops a powerful argument about the exclusion of vulnerable people in society. Ballatt and Campling go to the edges of kinship, where compassion may be difficult, where, for example, the immigration centre at Yarl's Wood was described by the children's commissioner as 'no place for a child'. When I was reading the chapters discussing older people in hospital and end-of-life care, I could feel for myself a despairing anger. I could very much identify with the issues in these chapters. They got to me, you could say. The section on organisational change, and the use the authors make of Susan Long's theory of organisational perversity, is also powerful, and I could wish that the modernisers would learn to be more reflective. But the message is not depressing. The authors engage the reader in an intense conversation. Intelligent kindness is never needed more than in end-of-life care, when there is a pressure to function as what Obholzer described as a 'keep death at bay' service.

Do not expect to agree with everything the authors say, but be prepared to enter into the argument. Some readers may think that all this is too much a polemic. Well, it is a polemic, and it may be that more and more readers have the stomach for robust criticism of the processes that destabilise good practice. The book is an important companion piece to the earlier work of Alyson Pollock and others on the changes in the National Health Service (NHS), where the marketisation and privatisation of services put constraints on the space for compassion.

The final section is a constructive examination and critique of the organisational and wider political issues. Underpinning this discussion are the ideas that compassion has to be part of a gift relationship and cannot be enforced, and that a lack of trust has desperate consequences, unassuaged by the myth of the perfect regulatory system.

The writers discuss a culture of coercive management, of turning a blind eye to self-evident faults in the delivery of care, and the increasing commodification of professional vocation (contrasted with the ordinary kindness of basic-grade workers). They describe the NHS under pressure and stress the need for calm and stability in the context of 're-disorganisation'. They show us how we may learn from some of the most powerful recent sources, including the report on Mid-Staffordshire NHS Foundation Trust, and explore the 'pull towards perversion', when a sense of priorities becomes confused in an industrialised, target-driven market economy encouraging the commodification of care. The fear is that the opening of NHS provision to any willing provider will accelerate this process.

The concluding discussion about intelligent kindness is constructive and encouraging. The people who will make the NHS work are the people who work in the NHS. In the context of the 'Big Society', the NHS is itself an expression of community, of reciprocity of need. Those who deliver health and social care deserve our best wishes. This book helps us to look to their needs if they are to respond to ours – with kindness.

Acknowledgements

We have been buoyed up by the interest and encouragement of friends and colleagues, especially Gwen Adshead, Sabyasachi Bhaumik, Christopher Campling, Paul Gilbert, Richard Jones, Piotr Kuhivchak, Liz Logie, Philippa Marx, Barrie Rathbone, Felicity Rosslyn and Graeme Whitfield. We are immensely grateful to Chris Maloney and Bob Palmer, who, as well as cheering us on, went the extra mile and offered critique, expertise, advice and material to help us frame and refine our argument and its presentation. Many others who have inspired us through our careers are well represented in the text.

Thanks also to Martin Fahy, Neil Doverty and Sabyasachi Bhaumik from the Leicestershire Partnership NHS Trust for generously supporting Penny's sabbatical – time which helped us shape this book and establish the momentum to keep going through busy times.

Close family and friends have warmed us on our way and coped kindly with our preoccupation: in particular, Natasha Davies, Debbie Chaloner and John Dent.

We owe particular gratitude to Bernard Ratigan and Jane Lawton for helping us keep our theme sensitively in mind.

Introduction

For over 60 years, the National Health Service (NHS) has been a central feature of British life. From the cradle to the grave, citizens are promised healthcare, delivered according to need, free at the point of delivery. We look to it to protect our health, to help us bring our children into the world, to treat our illnesses, from the trivial to the life-threatening, and to care for us in our time of dying. We pay for it, of course, through taxation and National Insurance contributions. On our behalf, the government sets the priorities and standards for the NHS and regulates it, and allocates our money to local organisations and clinicians to manage and deliver our care.

In our view, what is important at the root of this arrangement is that all citizens are taking responsibility for one another. The public *share* the risks of accident and illness, the costs of caring for each other, the responsibility for the limits to the resources, and for setting the priorities relating to how the NHS develops. Although it is large and complex, and in obvious ways like an industry, it is, we think, much more than that. It is a by-no-means perfect arrangement that invites society to value and attend to its deepest common interest and connectedness. It is an expression of community, and one that can improve (in terms of quality and efficiency) if society, patients and staff can reconnect to and be helped to realise these deeper values.

We are aware that valuing these aspects of the British approach to public healthcare is controversial and can attract vehement opposition. It is not surprising that throughout its history the NHS has evoked powerful feelings in citizens and staff (who are citizens too) of gratitude, pride and protectiveness, and also of concern, disappointment and anger. Of course, the venture was political, and remains so – and this opens up questions and evokes strong feelings. The mainstream political parties in the UK are currently committed, at least publicly, to the NHS, but the range of ideologies and methodologies of 'reform' or 'transformation' often chime uncomfortably with the intention and power of the underlying vision.

Whatever its denigrators have said, the NHS has worked. The chronic under-resourcing (compared with healthcare expenditure in other industrialised countries) through the last decades of the 20th century had a detrimental effect on treatments and outcomes for some conditions, but the country's overall health statistics in the second part of the 20th century compared well with those of similar countries (Pollack, 2004, pp. 40–41). Life expectancy remained consistently above the US and EU average and infant mortality rates were consistently lower, despite the fact that healthcare expenditure per capita was much less than the US or EU average and the UK spent much less on health as a percentage of gross domestic product (GDP), according to the Office of Health Economics (see Pollock, 2004, p. 35).

The Labour government brought spending up to the European average between 2002 and 2007, with large-scale increases in workforce, improved access to services and shorter waiting times, during a period when demand increased significantly. NHS healthcare environments improved, though by no means universally. Criticisms that this increased funding did not yield sufficient impact may hold water. Much of the investment found its way into pay awards, Private Finance Initiatives, reorganisations and successive forms of regulation and commissioning. But that is a criticism of government strategy, not of the NHS. Although the Conservative–Liberal Democrat coalition government since May 2010 has made much of poor comparisons between some health outcomes in the UK and those in some other industrialised countries, the trend of improvement shows that the NHS will soon equal or overtake their performance. This is true even though the UK spends 2.5 percentage points less of its GDP on healthcare than does, for example, France (Appleby, 2011).

Let us accept from the start that no approach is perfect. Individuals do face limits to what the state, husbanding limited resources on our joint behalf, will and can fund – whether it be new drugs or treatments, new hospitals or more staffing. A universal, comprehensive, system requires steering, commissioning, regulating and managing on a grand scale. The system can foster unhelpful dependency and a lack of personal responsibility for health. Citizens, and workers within the NHS, can both develop a sense of passive (and sometimes aggressive) entitlement to their services or ways of working and jobs.

Priorities are often hard to agree on, especially with the rapid rise in the ageing population and with the development of new treatments and health technologies, and even harder to reconcile locally. These priorities can be skewed by public panic, interest groups who shout loudest, ideas about most (and least) deserving groups, media campaigns, stigma and denial. Our public investment in healthcare can be vulnerable to wider events – war, recession, crime and the costs of other public priorities. Just how much, anyway, should we, as a population, require our government to invest on our behalf in health and healthcare? Up to what standards and with what priorities? How much tax are we willing to pay in any case? The continued existence of the NHS depends on voters being confident that it is worth their while to invest their 'healthcare insurance' in taxes – and this is hard to judge, both for individuals and for society.

Nonetheless, we believe that the NHS is the best way to go about securing the healthcare of a civilised society. Struggling with the inevitable difficulties in such a model is worth it. It means universal free access to healthcare and a commitment to the ethical and systematic organisation of resources to provide it. But it also embodies society's pooled investment in its collective well-being, shared risk and shared responsibility for each other, making the NHS one of the most socially valuable of all institutions. Although our book focuses on UK healthcare, many of the ideas we explore are, we believe, applicable beyond that arena – to healthcare systems in other countries, and to social care.

We have worked in the NHS – in clinical and leadership roles – for many years. We have cared for people, supervised and trained staff, managed budgets, delivered savings and reshaped services. We have developed strategy and managed change. In our work, we have made mistakes and done things we are proud of. We have been patients, needing care and services from many parts of the healthcare system at different times in our lives. We have supported children, friends and elderly relatives through healthcare at times of accident, illness and dying. We have had varied experiences in all these roles – some apparently relating to 'the system' and some to the attitudes and skills of staff. It has frequently been difficult to tell the difference.

We accept that the project of delivering an efficient, effective and high-quality NHS requires a form of management that will inevitably include a range of ideologies and techniques. The scale and elaborateness of the approach, the models and methods used, and the way services are led and managed require careful judgement. Despite their successes, we have not, overall, been impressed by many of the realities of the implementation of the Labour government's 'reform' project and fear that changes under the coalition government's Health and Social Care Bill will undermine the NHS even further.

More importantly, we are concerned that so little attention has been given to understanding and promoting what we see as central to the NHS enterprise as a whole: its embodiment of *kinship*, and its expression in the *compassionate relationship* between the skilled clinician and the patient. To fail to attend to the promotion of kinship, connectedness and kindness between staff and with patients is to fail to address a key dimension of what makes people do well for others. Such failures can sometimes be no more than minor irritations, but they can lead to appalling systemic abuses, neglect and maltreatment – as evidenced in successive reports of inquiries into the care of the elderly (Health Services Ombudsman, 2011), people with intellectual disabilities (Michael, 2008) and several acute healthcare trusts (Healthcare Commission, 2007, 2009). All such scandals immediately raise in the public mind disturbing questions about how compassion can fail. And yet that question receives far less attention in subsequent corrective action than it deserves. We think these questions require much more thorough investigation. Abuses can, and do, happen in public and private healthcare services: the exploration in this book seeks to shed light on some of the factors leading to failures in compassion, especially in the NHS in the UK.

The absence of attention to the question of kindness is particularly disturbing because we see the NHS project itself as an expression of kinship and common interest in the face of risk, danger and death. What is more likely to ensure that everybody strives to make it work than paying attention to how to engage people in that value-based vision and supporting them in making it real? What is more likely to motivate people to address inequalities and to champion people's rights?

We believe that putting a fraction of the effort that has gone into processes of organising, regulating and industrialising the NHS into developing our understanding of what helps and hinders kindness in its staff would have enormous ramifications for effectiveness and efficiency, as well as for the experience of the patient. If we were to apply that understanding intelligently to the way we run things, our public hopes and expectations for the service would be far more likely to be met. It may be unavoidable that we have, some of the time, to consider and frame healthcare from a transactional, commodified, industrial and value-for-money perspective. We argue, however, that to undervalue attention to NHS healthcare as a commitment to the skilled and effective expression of fellow feeling and kindness, through the relationship between staff and patient, is dangerous. It will lead to waste and poor performance, to low morale and poor patient satisfaction, to continued shameful abuses.

There is, perhaps surprisingly, a substantial body of knowledge to shed light on the subject of what kindness is, and what managing to be kind is about. This knowledge relates to the attitudes and behaviour of individuals, to teams and groups, to organisations and to society. It illuminates our understanding of why things go wrong, of why people behave unkindly, and also what conditions promote kindness and consequent well-being. It shows direct links between kindness and effectiveness and positive outcomes. It suggests virtuous circles where kindness promotes well-being, reduces stress and increases satisfaction for the patient, the worker and the organisation.

We are not suggesting yet another labyrinthine 'national programme'. Nor are we proposing some sentimental crusade. We do not advocate a 'technology of kindness'. But what if this body of knowledge were to be used to develop our understanding about how to reform, improve and ensure the quality and value for money of health services? What if we understood better how to bring out, nurture and protect kindness and its related attentiveness to what others need? What if people were educated, trained and managed to bring this understanding into practice, whether as policy makers, managers or clinical staff?

This book is an experiment with this approach. We hope it offers an impetus to the process of mustering the knowledge, arguments and evidence to develop this alternative view of reform. We hope it will go some way to justify priority being given to tempering the more mechanical and industrial reform programme through the intelligent promotion of kindness.

Our book is not an attempt to provide an encyclopaedic coverage of the subject. The aim is to offer sufficient argument and illustration, to raise questions and to indicate further directions for the general reader, for student clinicians and practitioners, and for people working in healthcare at every level. To develop the paradigm that we imagine would need the collaboration of a lot of people – just as the elaborate regulation and structural change agenda has required. They exist – the specialists in various forms of knowledge and skills, and the ordinary (and extraordinary) people working in the system who, we believe, would thrive better were they to be invited into ways of working indicated by an understanding of kindness. If our book can engage people's curiosity, promote some confidence that the approach is worth pursuing and sketch some of the landscape that requires exploring, we will have achieved our purpose. We should say from the start that we believe passionately in the NHS, and know that there is much that is excellent, kind and effective in the work of the 1.3 million staff who contribute their intelligence, skills and effort. If we address some of its problems and failures directly, it is to advance our argument that there is a way of dealing with them based on applying what can be understood about kindness. We do not want to denigrate the widespread excellence of the work of hosts of dedicated people.

This book is *not* about sentimental niceness or simple altruism. As our opening chapter will attest, kindness is something that is generated by an intellectual and emotional understanding that *self-interest and the interests of others are bound together,* and by acting upon that understanding. Human beings have enormous capacity for kindness, but also for destructiveness and violence. We make no apology for spending time examining some of the roots and causes of *unkindness,* with a view to illuminating how best to promote and nourish kindness in the work of healthcare staff. Whether politics are striving to create the Big Society, the Good Society, or any other vision of national well-being, the strategies adopted will mean little unless they promote positive emotional engagement and the intelligent application of skills and resources, to manage darker impulses well.

Aspects of kindness appear in various forms across healthcare policy in the UK, which is to be celebrated. There is, though, a frequent sense that it is the junior partner alongside other ideologies and goals, leaning over the shoulder of more important things. Whether kindness is helped or hindered by these other aspects of policy and reform is seldom considered. We aim to bring kindness into the foreground in the crowded company of policies and technologies for NHS reform and to do it the justice of examining some of the ways it is helped and hindered by its fellows.

Finally, a note on our use of words. We have chosen to use the expression 'patient' throughout this book. This is because we want to stress the link with compassion – a patient is someone we 'feel (or even suffer) with'. We are aware that the focus on suffering could be regarded as reinforcing the unhelpful idea that patients are passive victims – but we believe that people's strengths are more readily inspired when they feel that their suffering is recognised and understood. We are all patients – of our general practitioners at the very least – whether we are ill or not, whether we 'use services' or not. Citizens may, rightly, need the power to exercise choice, even, at times, to be empowered as 'customers', but, above all, they need and deserve a compassionate, skilled response to their suffering.

References

Appleby J. (2011) Data briefing. Does poor health justify NHS reform? *BMJ*, **342**, d566.

Healthcare Commission (2007) *The Investigation Report into* Clostridium difficile *at Maidstone and Tunbridge Wells NHS Trust*. HMSO.

Healthcare Commission (2009) *The Investigation into Mid Staffordshire NHS Foundation Trust*. Healthcare Commission.

Health Services Ombudsman (2011) *Care and Compassion? A Report of the Health Services Ombudsman on Ten Investigations into NHS Care for Older People*. HMSO.

Michael, J. (2008) *Healthcare for All: Report of the Independent Inquiry into Access to Healthcare For People With Learning Disabilities*. HMSO.

Pollock, A. M. (2004) *NHS plc: The Privatisation of Our Health Care*. Verso.

Part I
Healthy kindness

CHAPTER 1

Rescuing kindness

Yet do I fear thy nature; it is too full o' the milk of human kindness.
(William Shakespeare, *Macbeth*)

Kindness and kinship

The word 'kindness' evokes mixed feelings in the modern world. To begin this exploration of its importance and value in transforming healthcare, it is important to bring into focus what it is we are discussing. This means attempting a definition. Almost more importantly, it means rescuing the concept (and what it indicates) from the grip of a range of social and cultural forces that warp, denigrate and obscure what it is, marginalise kindness in the debate about what matters, and make it more difficult to be kind.

As an adjective, *kind* means being of a sympathetic, helpful or forbearing nature and, importantly for our subject, being inclined to bring pleasure or relief. It is important to keep it rooted in its deeper meanings, though. It can easily become a mere synonym for individual acts of generosity, sentiment and affection, for a general, fuzzy 'kindliness'. The Old English noun *cynd* metamorphosed through Middle English to become *kinde* and into our modern language as *kind*. The word meant 'nature', 'family', 'lineage' – 'kin'. It indicated what we are, who we are and that we are linked together, in the present and across time.

The word *kindness* indicates the quality or state of being kind. It describes a condition in which people recognise their nature, know and feel that this is essentially one with that of their kin, understand and feel their interdependence, feel responsibility for their successors and express all this in attitudes and actions towards each other. Kindness is both an obligation to one's kin born of our understanding of our connectedness, and the natural expression of our attitudes and feelings arising from this connectedness. Real acts of kindness emerge from this state. Kindness challenges us to be self-aware and takes us to the heart of relationships, where things can be messy, difficult and painful. It is closely linked with the concept of compassion (literally, suffering with), sympathy (fellow feeling) and the biblical word *agape* (neighbourly or 'brotherly' love). People who are 'rooted' in a sense of kinship with each other are inclined to attentiveness to the other, to gentleness, warmth and creativity on their behalf. Kindness is kinship felt and expressed.

Kindness is natural – we see it all around us. It drives people to pay attention to each other, to try to understand what they enjoy, what they need. It emerges from a sense of common humanity, promotes sharing, effort on others' behalf, sacrifice for the good of the other. It drives imagination, resourcefulness and creativity in interpersonal, family, community and international life. When people are kind, they want to do well for others. It is also difficult, involving overcoming narrow self-interest, anxiety, conflict, distaste and limited resources. Kindness involves the risk of getting things wrong, maybe of being hurt somehow in the process. Kindness is most effective when directed by intelligence. It really is no good fixing the boiler for the elderly lady next door if you are not qualified in gas engineering, however good she or you feel about your apparent generosity. Knowing not to feed a hungry newborn with pasta can be a help. Understanding the challenges of adolescence can lead to more productive, and less exhausting, parenting.

Kindness is necessary, too, in general and special forms. Most decorated service personnel directly ascribe their heroism to strong, intimate fellow feeling and kinship with their comrades – as individuals and as groups. They know and feel that they are 'kin', 'of a kind', and act accordingly. Such inspiring connectedness is also required when a parent cleans the faeces and vomit of the infant or when the clinical worker sees through frightening, distasteful evidence of accident or illness to care for the person suffering. The armed services, along with their emphasis on drill, discipline and chain of command, put enormous effort and skill into promoting connectedness, loyalty and kinship. This fellow feeling helps those in the services to overcome fear, focus on their frightening task and work together – even in the face of death.

It cannot be said that the same attention is given to the promotion of fellow feeling and kinship in the NHS, and that is alarming. It is particularly worrying because NHS staff need not only to develop solidarity among themselves against a common enemy. They must work together to meet others (patients and their families), to connect with them, ascertain their needs (which is frequently difficult), treat them and help them stay well. There is something rather distasteful about the current vogue for the metaphor of 'war' in health – the 'war' on cancer was much promoted in late 2009, for example. However, clinicians and patients occupy a field full of dangers, uncertainties and choices that frequently demand teamwork in crisis, courage and intense relationship. Daily life is full of routine, procedures and resources that need to be brought to life and marshalled to address real needs and dangers for real human beings. Though the risk to the clinician is far less overtly dramatic than that to the soldier, there are frequent high risks of mistakes, of things going wrong, of illness killing the patient. Small errors can have enormous consequences. To fail to attend to promoting kinship, connectedness and kindness between staff and with patients is to fail to address a key dimension of what makes people do well for others in such circumstances.

For centuries, kindness was seen as a primary virtue. Critically, that does not mean it was simply regarded as 'a good thing'. A virtue has to be worked at, because achieving it is, however 'natural', difficult. All major religions, and the cultures they have influenced, promote compassion, hospitality to the stranger, treating other people as one would wish to be treated oneself, indeed 'loving kindness', within a recognition that much of human nature pushes against it (Armstrong, 2009). But kindness as we have defined it is not just asserted as a virtue in religion. It has also had a central place in secular – indeed materialist – movements.

Political concepts such as the brotherhood of 'man', socialism and other revolutionary movements, and projects such as anti-slavery, women's suffrage and anti-racism are all centred on the idea of overcoming apparent differences, removing conditions of inequality, disadvantage and suffering, restoring kinship. Right-wing movements are also characterised by an idea of kinship – of a folk, a family, a race, a nation. Here, though, we see 'kinship' being defined *against* or *at the expense of* rather than *including* and *in the interests of* others. Such a position is also readily identifiable in the more fundamentalist religious movements, which set themselves and their kin against those of other religions and of none. In left thinking, too, especially revolutionary socialism, a principle that we are all equal and interdependent, a commitment to serving the common interest ('from each according to their ability; to each according to their need') has nevertheless frequently split 'the human family' into insiders and outsiders.

One of the more problematic aspects to kinship, then, is whom we include as kin, and how we understand and manage the difficulties in our relationships and obligations 'within the family' and 'with the other'. How we behave on that boundary determines how much kinship is expressed as kindness beyond narrow self-interest.

That the espousal of the virtue has been used to justify all sorts of means, ranging from the inspired to the barbaric, in both religious and secular life, shows, of course, that a philosophical attachment to kindness is not enough. Kindness implies an attitude of openheartedness and generosity, but also a *practice* that can be challenging and risky and that requires *skill*. The inconsistency in the true application of the virtue has not just been because it is hard to fight unkindness in the world: it is also because it can be very hard to be kind, individually or in groups. That, in turn, is hard to admit.

Kindness disparaged

A consequence of this has been a growing tendency to suspect any person, movement or institution promoting kindness as naïve, hopelessly idealistic and ineffectual, or even sinister, hypocritical and dangerous. We have learned to suspect assertions of values like kindness and kinship, and to put our faith into more selfish, technical, more 'privatised' things. In modern Western society this retreat from kinship has been accelerated by a wide range of powerful influences.

The warping and obscuring of what kindness is about have been extensively discussed by psychoanalyst Adam Phillips and historian Barbara Taylor in their book *On Kindness* (2009). They explore the way in which a philosophy and culture of competitive individualism and the pursuance of self-interest have challenged the value, and negatively influenced the meaning, of kindness. Kindness, they say, is not a temptation to sacrifice ourselves, but to include ourselves with others – kindness is being in solidarity with human need. They describe a process in which what had been a core moral value, with a subversive edge, at centre stage in the political battles of the Enlightenment, became something sentimentalised, marginalised and denigrated through the 19th and into the early 20th century:

Kindness was steadily downgraded from a universal imperative to the prerogative of specific social constituencies: romantic poets, clergymen, charity-workers and above all, women, whose presumed tender-heartedness survived the egoist onslaught. By the end of the Victorian period, kindness had been largely feminized, ghetto-ized into a womanly sphere of feeling and behaviour where it has remained, with some notable exceptions, ever since. (Phillips & Taylor, 2009, p. 41)

Gradually, the value and pertinence of kindness was edged into this periphery by a spirit of 'manly' rugged individualism and competitive enterprise. This movement was closely associated with the Industrial Revolution, with its valuing of scientific progress, technology and entrepreneurship, reinforced by the attitudes and wars of Empire. A split developed between (empty-headed, unrealistic, amateur, female) kindness and (knowing, clear-sighted, professional, male) competitive enterprise and the pursuit of self-interest. A range of other cultural crowbars reinforced this split. One of the key influences was that of mass production and the associated market. This increasingly shifted the emphasis in people's lives to being consumers rather than sharers, to acquisition and to the competitiveness that used quaintly to be referred to as 'keeping up with the Jones's' and might today be expressed as keeping up with the Americans or Chinese.

Increasingly, this quest for security and well-being through acquisitiveness and material goods has centred on technology and industry – as possession, as that which makes and secures these possessions, and that which communicates and displays them. Such competitiveness is not reserved for wealth and possessions but extends into all aspects of social life. This is most vivid in celebrity culture and the myriad 'reality television' shows that tout their popularity (and the reverse) with the public, or that offer 'wannabes' the chance to join the celebrity family. To return to Phillips & Taylor:

A culture of 'hardness' and cynicism grows, fed by envious admiration of those who seem to thrive – the rich and famous: our modern priesthood – in this tooth-and-claw environment. (p. 108)

An individualistic, competitive society, is, then, whatever its achievements, prone to breed unkindness.

Kindness and survival

A strong driver of the imbalance towards competitiveness and self-interest has been a widespread misapplication – and misrepresentation – of social Darwinism, which has had increasing influence in economics, politics and most aspects of social life. Competition, based on self-interest, has been reinforced by ideas derived from simplistic readings of Darwinism itself – the skewed reading of nature as 'red in tooth and claw'. Later work, such as Richard Dawkins' *The Selfish Gene* (Dawkins, 1976), has fed such a rhetoric and been used as an 'evidence base' for justifying the promotion of competition and individualism in politics and economics, as well as in social and personal life. Nowhere is this influence more evident than in the way 'free market forces' (the unregulated competitive interaction of enterprises bent on self-interest) have been regarded, until very recently, as benign, creative and even natural – indeed, as the only road to human well-being.

In fact, Dawkins is clear that reciprocity based on a sense of human kinship is an evolutionary reality. Action directed even by the most 'selfish' of genes is expressly characterised by the fact that its interests lie in caring for others who carry that same gene – kinship. Dawkins is also passionate about our unique (evolved) capacity as human beings to transcend the purely determined and to transform civilisation using our intelligence and moral consciousness (Dawkins, 2009). Other students of evolution have recognised that Darwin himself described an important role for cooperation and interdependence in *The Origin of Species* (1859). Many scientists, including, notably Lynn Margulis, have described a remarkably powerful place for cooperation within and between species in evolution itself (Margulis, 1998). Kinship and its expression in kindness can, then, be seen not just as a psychosocial concept, but as the representation in human psychology and social life of a primary evolutionary process.

When apes descended from the trees and began to evolve into us, competitive tool-making helped, but cooperation and kinship transformed and combined the invention and ingenuity of individuals into a social evolutionary force of unimaginable power. Cooperation actually creates 'the fittest' who 'survive'. Reproductive success may have been dependent on having the most impressive tools, but it was through sharing them that the conditions emerged for accelerated development to increased safety and comfort. This sharing, at least at the level of higher animals and primates, is clearly driven in everyday interaction by recognition of the other, and their well-being, as connected, as in specific need and as deserving assistance. This idea, and the kindness involved at a human level, needs to be restored to its rightful place.

Enterprise, self-confidence and self-reliance, individualism and science and technology are all of value. It is the *split* between these qualities and those of kinship and interdependency that is disturbing. Without the recognition, and balancing influence, of common destiny and connectedness inherent in kindness, these things can become toxic. The unregulated financial market, the fetishism of the body as a commodity or building site for 'beauty', and unrestrained polluting industry are various forms of this toxin. Social well-being degenerates as these products of the split multiply. Without applying our knowledge of the power of cooperation, inspired by kinship and expressed through kindness, we will fail to create the thriving society most would look for. We are all, more than ever, interdependent at a planetary level, and our future depends on our being able to cooperate – and better than we have ever done before. Moreover, global issues, such as climate change, challenge us to be imaginative enough to extend our sense of kinship to generations as yet unborn, as well as to other countries, such as Bangladesh and Pakistan, where the crisis is already extreme.

The trouble with kindness

Apart from universal human struggles to overcome self-centredness, bad temper and greed (daunting in themselves) there is a deeper problem associated with kindness. As Phillips & Taylor (2009) put it:

Real kindness changes people in the doing of it, often in unpredictable ways. Real kindness is an exchange with essentially unpredictable consequences. It is a risk precisely because it mingles our needs and desires with the needs and desires of others, in a way that so-called self-interest never can. (p. 12)

Kindness, then, is, deep down, frightening and hazardous.

In the modern world, this problem with kindness is particularly challeng-ing. The risks to health and well-being in genetics, lifestyle, relationships, society, environment and international affairs are more than ever known, by more and more of us. There is clear evidence that anxiety levels (or their twin, attitudes of denial) are consequently higher. Education and the media also bring us all increased exposure to the vulnerability, suffering and dangerousness of humankind, close to home and afar. We are daily confronted with evidence of just how perilous it is to link ourselves with the destiny of others. This all goes to amplify the danger inherent in kindness and cooperation. It takes courage to link one's fate with others with vast and frightening problems.

Phillips & Taylor, quoted above, speak of kindness being 'ghetto-ized into a ... sphere of feeling and behaviour where it has remained, with some notable exceptions, ever since' (p. 41). The foundation of the NHS was one of those notable exceptions – as well as being an optimistic project to eradicate ill health, it was an expression of kinship, a commitment to kindness.

In the Second World War, British men and women had laboured for each other, fought, been wounded, bereaved and died for the sake of the common good. The founding of the NHS after the war saw a peacetime expression of this commitment. At one and the same time it was an act of appreciation and recognition by the people to the people, and a compact and understanding between us that we would continue to share our resources to face our common risks and improve our common destiny. It was an expression of *kinship*. We took our vulnerability, woundedness and loss, our courage, self-sacrifice and fellow feeling, and invested them, along with our resources and our ingenuity, in a peacetime 'family enterprise'. Like war, this common pursuit would bring us, individually and collectively, victories and defeats, costs and advantages, miracles and tragedies.

Phillips & Taylor argue that this commitment to communal well-being was, in fact, short-lived. They suggest that the individualism, independence and 'enterprise culture' that has emerged over the past 30 years or so has been a very poor soil for the growth of kindness. On the other hand, signs of the founding values of the NHS can still be detected and it is central to our argument that the NHS should be valued as a core aspect of our public good, which goes further than improving health and treating sickness. Take a look at the 2009 NHS Constitution for England:

The NHS belongs to the people. It is there to improve our health and well-being, supporting us to keep mentally and physically well, to get better when we are ill, and, when we cannot fully recover, to stay as we can to the end of our lives. ... It touches our lives at times of basic human need, when care and compassion are what matters most. ... The NHS is founded on a common set of principles and values that bind together the community and the people it serves – patients and public – and the staff who work for it. (Department of Health, 2009, p. 2)

This document commits the NHS to work in partnership to prevent ill health, to provide care that is personal, effective and safe. The policy also sets down the latest expression of values of the NHS: respect and dignity, commitment to quality of care, compassion, improving lives, working together for patients and 'everyone counting'. It is evident that the NHS is still seen as having a responsibility to deliver on the public compact of communal kindness that is identified as its foundation. There are, though, problems in translating that view into action.

Given the sustained onslaught on the value and power of kindness, the untrammelled growth of the culture of self-interest and the deep fears kindness evokes, it is unsurprising that all of us – from citizen to government – lose our nerve. At times of stretched resources – like the current effects of recession – this loss of nerve is more likely. Instead of valuing and reinforcing the core kinship and kindness involved in the health service, we become like the Puritans of old, with no sense that pursuing the health and happiness of others is an inherent pleasure for individuals and society. We turn our minds to setting rules for and to policing people we seem not to trust. At best, we appear to prefer to think of this enterprise mainly in terms of technology, industrial systems, processes, survival statistics, financial efficiency and 'rights'. Could it be that we have all lost confidence? Could it be that we have all succumbed to anxiety and embarrassment about focusing on the central vision of kinship, the reciprocity and the values it requires? Could it be that we have lost confidence in the idea that keeping connected to that vision can make a difference?

All of us may have lost our nerve in this way; all of us, that is, except when we or our loved ones are patients. Then the importance of kindness comes to the centre of things. Patients realise how kindness makes them feel. Just as important, they seem to know how closely it is connected to effectiveness.

Kindness and the common good

Kindness, then, is not a soft, sentimental feeling or action that is beside the point in the challenging, clever, technical business of managing and delivering healthcare. It is a binding, creative and problem-solving force that inspires and focuses the imagination and goodwill. It inspires and directs the attention and efforts of people and organisations towards building relationships with patients, recognising their needs and treating them well. Kindness is not a 'nice' side issue in the project of competitive progress. It is the 'glue' of cooperation required for such progress to be of most benefit to most people.

The mistrust that has been evoked in society relating to the motives and behaviours of those professing to be kind was highlighted earlier. The concept of kindness in this book assumes authenticity, where emotional response and behaviour are in tune and spring from generosity, empathy and openheartedness. This rules out those whose seemingly kind bedside manner masks sadistic motives and behaviour – Harold Shipman being the most extreme example – and those who preach kindness as a duty but are unable to connect genuinely with the living humanity of another person. It also rules out those who gush with sentiment; and the self-righteously pious, whose primary motivation is to be saintly.

There is no doubt that kindness, though it makes us all feel better, is difficult. Later chapters will discuss the nature of this difficulty and consider some of the ways in which it can be overcome. But from the start, we need to make sure we are comfortable with, and properly understand, the concept of kindness itself. The renowned academic historian Tony Judt wrote passionately about collective welfare and the values of community (Judt, 2010a). In an interview just before he died, he spoke movingly about the need for a language that binds us all together:

We need to rediscover a language of dissent. It can't be an economic language since part of the problem is that we have for too long spoken about politics in an economic language where everything has been about growth, efficiency, productivity and wealth, and not enough has been about collective ideals around which we can gather, around which we can get angry together, around which we can be motivated collectively, whether on the issue of justice, inequality, cruelty or unethical behaviour. We have thrown away the language with which to do that. And until we rediscover that language how could we possibly bind ourselves together? (Judt, 2010b).

Fundamental to this project are questions about kindness: whether we dare rescue the enlightened concept of kindness, with its depth and political potency, whether we can find a way to use it to edge us towards a society based on the common good, and whether we can unashamedly re-own the language of kinship and the simplicity with which it asserts our common humanity. Nowhere is this more important than in healthcare.

References

Armstrong, K. (2009) Charter for Compassion. See http://charterforcompassion.org (last accessed March 2011).

Darwin, C. (1859) *On the Origin of Species*. John Murray.

Dawkins, R. (1976) *The Selfish Gene*. Oxford University Press.

Dawkins, R. (2009) *The Genius of Charles Darwin* (DVD). Channel 4.

Department of Health (2009) *The NHS Constitution for England: The NHS Belongs To Us All*. HMSO.

Judt, T. (2010a) *Ill Fares the Land: A Treatise on Our Present Discontents*. Allen Lane.

Judt, T. (2010b) Interviewed in *London Review of Books*, 25 March.

Margulis, L. (1998) *Symbiotic Planet: A New Look At Evolution*. Orion Books.

Phillips, A. & Taylor, P. (2009) *On Kindness*. Penguin.

CHAPTER 2

A politics of kindness

No injustice is greater than the inequalities in health which scar our nation. (Department of Health, 2000)

To dare to look at the NHS through the prism of what we know about kindness requires, of course, strong justification. In short, the argument is that focusing on kinship expressed through kindness will improve health and healthcare, and, indeed, efficiency. Some of the supporting evidence is found before we even open the door to the consulting room or the hospital, or follow the community nurse into a patient's home. It relates to the dynamics of kinship at a societal and political level.

Poverty and health

Improvements in the health of a nation are due to many things other than the way it chooses to organise healthcare delivery. While there is no doubt that the health of the population improved during the early years of the NHS, the reasons for this were many. These included medical advances such as the use of antibiotics and vaccination programmes. However, socioeconomic factors clearly played a significant role in improvements in general health, particularly the lessening of absolute poverty, which, in the UK in the last century, was addressed through the financial safety nets and supports of the welfare state. Much of the progress was a continuation of a process of sanitary reform that began in the 19th century. The early decades of the NHS coincided with a period known by public health specialists as the *epidemiological transition*, when infectious diseases lost their hold as the major cause of death in the industrialised world. Chronic diseases such as heart disease and cancer replaced infections as the main cause of mortality. Though the toll of these diseases is serious, the general levels of health in the higher-income countries have been rising for some time.

The link between poverty and poor health is well known; the fact that people at the bottom of society have shorter lives and suffer more illness is no surprise (Department of Health, 2009). The World Health Organization's Commission on Social Determinants of Health published a hard-hitting report in 2008 with the stark message that, on a global perspective, *social injustice is killing people on a grand scale*. In Britain, health disparities have been a major item on the public health agenda for years, with at least a 7-year difference in life expectancy between the lowest and highest socio-economic groups. The Marmot review, *Fair Society: Healthy Lives* (Marmot, 2010), advocates reducing health inequalities through putting social justice, health and sustainability at the heart of all policies. The report is critical of the poor record of policy in tackling health inequalities in the UK and places an emphasis on delivery systems and leadership. Sadly, the report confirms that the health gap between the average and worse-off areas is wider than it was in 1997. Moreover, it is not simply a matter of the poor having worse health than everyone else: in richer countries, higher incomes are related to a lower death rate at every level of society.

If we look a bit deeper at what was going on in Britain in the years preceding the foundation of the NHS, some interesting issues emerge. In the two decades between the world wars, the increase in life expectancy for civilians was 6–7 years for men and women. This is roughly *twice* that seen throughout the rest of the 20th century in the eight decades before and after the wars, where the increase in life expectancy was between 1 and 4 years (Wilkinson, 1996). This is surprising given the fact that material living standards declined during both wars. It is true that nutritional status improved with rationing in the 1940s, but rationing continued into the 1950s and did not happen during the First World War. Both periods of war were characterised, however, by full employment and narrower income differences, and rates of relative poverty were halved. Could it be that the encouragement to cooperate with the war effort, the reduction in inequality, the resulting sense of mutuality, camaraderie and kindness contributed in some way to better health?

Income inequality also appears to have a dramatic effect on the health of a nation. In Japan after the Second World War, the huge redistribution of wealth and power led to an egalitarian economy with unrivalled improvement in population health (Subramanian & Kawachi, 2004). In contrast, Russia has experienced dramatic decreases in life expectancy since the early 1990s as it has moved from a centrally planned to a market economy, accompanied by a rapid rise in income inequality (Walberg *et al*, 1998). Perhaps the best-known example is that of impoverished and egalitarian Cuba, which has lower infant mortality rates than its rich neighbour, the USA, and a similar life expectancy to the UK (Hertzman *et al*, 2010).

Public health, it seems, is improved not only by reductions in absolute poverty, but also by the strength of the shared motives and connections between people and the degree of income equality. This has been referred to as 'the big idea', and while it is an idea that attracts passionate opposition, the evidence supporting it continues to accumulate (*BMJ*, 1996; Pickett & Wilkinson, 2009).

Inequality and health outcomes

In their book *The Spirit Level*, Richard Wilkinson & Kate Pickett (2009) collate the evidence that inequalities are as crucial as absolute poverty in predicting the condition of a society, including the health of the population. Using 30 years of research data, they demonstrate that almost every modern social and environmental problem – ill health, breakdown of community life, violence, drug addiction, teenage births, obesity, mental illness, big prison populations and lack of social mobility – is more likely to occur in a less equal society. This appears to hold across all societies. Inequality is bad for poor countries because fewer people will have their basic needs met – access to clean water, food and shelter. In rich countries, where meeting such basic needs can generally be taken for granted and levels of absolute poverty are very low indeed, the effects of inequality are more complicated.

Examination of the relationship between life expectancy and national income per person shows life expectancy increasing rapidly with stage of economic development among poorer countries but this slows down and then levels off completely across the richest 30 or so countries (Wilkinson & Pickett, 2009, p. 7). Rates of economic growth are no longer linked to improving the general health of the population, which is now more to do with influencing lifestyle choices and managing risk. Among richer countries, the more unequal ones do worse even if they are richer overall, so that per capita GDP turns out to be much less significant for general well-being than the size of the gap between the richest and poorest 20% of the population (the basic measure of inequality the authors use).

What matters is the scale of material differences between people. In a country where the extent of material difference is low, the average life expectancy is likely to be higher and infant mortality rates lower than in a country where the gradient of material inequality is steeper. Comparisons between states in the USA also show this pattern, with unequal states clustering together regardless of income. Utah (relatively poor and equal) does as well as New Hampshire (relatively rich and equal) on a range of measures, while California (relatively rich and unequal) scores badly, like Mississippi (relatively poor and unequal) (Wilkinson & Pickett, 2009, pp. 22, 83).

The links between average health outcomes and income inequality in rich countries are strong across a range of health measures, in addition to life expectancy, as demonstrated by over 200 peer-reviewed studies of these associations (Kondo *et al*, 2009). It is not, though, simply the case that inequality means bad outcomes for those at the bottom of the social ladder. The link between inequality and poor health outcome is distributed across the social scale: it affects nearly everyone. What seems to matter is where you sit on the socioeconomic gradient in relation to other people within the same country, as well as the steepness of this gradient compared with the steepness of the gradient in other countries. How could this be? And does it have any link with kindness?

Chronic stress, inequality and health

Wilkinson and Pickett – and many others – have hypothesised that the link between equality and health is mediated through psychosocial mechanisms. In other words, material inequalities have a detrimental influence on social relations, which in turn affect people's psychological state, and physiological balance, particularly through the effects of chronic stress.

As affluent countries have grown richer, rates of anxiety and depression have risen, presumably as a result of the psychological and social effects of wealth, inequality and consumerism. Once a country has reached the level where a rise in average income makes no significant improvement to health and well-being, what purchases mean and say about status and identity is often more important than the goods themselves. Citizens are then caught in a stressful play of desire, uncertainty and choice. There is a growing literature about the tyranny of consumerism, the problematic nature of excessive choice and the stress this causes, in relatively wealthy societies. The American psychologist Barry Schwartz has explored this issue in such books as *The Paradox of Choice: Why More Is Less* (Schwartz, 2004).

Schwarz suggests (and uses research to demonstrate) that excessive choice evokes *paralysis*: too much choice makes choosing harder, promotes procrastination and lessens the likelihood of any choice being made. The enormous pressure put on the consumer by marketing on the basis of what goods say about you, combined with the technological complexity of those goods, promotes *high anxiety*. Choice increases that anxiety. He goes on to suggest that excessive choice evokes *dissatisfaction*. Choosing one thing from too wide a range of choices, finding any (inevitable) shortcoming, or later hearing (or dreaming) about some superior benefits of other options, leads to regret and reduced satisfaction with one's choice. This dissatisfaction fuels the anxiety that other choices are closed by the ones you make, or would be somehow better. Next, Schwartz argues that too much choice provokes an *escalation of expectations*: the quest for perfection is aroused, which, inevitably, amplifies dissatisfaction with both the choice you make and the range available.

This combination of paralysis, anxiety, dissatisfaction, disappointment and perfectionism is a fertile breeding ground for depression. Rich and poor alike are vulnerable to its effects as individuals. But the severity of this stress, and the degree to which it leads to depression (which is itself highly correlated with many physical conditions), appears to be very significantly influenced by relative inequality.

That the stress Schwartz describes is amplified by inequality may well be because people are preoccupied with status, image and possessions, and constantly driven to compare themselves to those around them. Even those with high incomes are likely to be more fearful of the repercussions of dropping down the social ladder than their counterparts in more egalitarian societies. Those 'beneath' them will be more preoccupied with their relative deprivation compared with the group above. As the economist Richard Layard put it, 'the consumption of the rich reduces everyone's satisfaction with what they have' (Layard, 2005, p. 53).

Modern life is stressful in so many ways – competitiveness (as expressed by longer working hours, higher debts, a greater percentage of GDP spent on advertising), uncertainty about the future, isolation and loneliness, worries about identity, lack of trust, too much choice, a risk-averse and high-blame culture. All these stresses are amplified where there are big differences between the haves and have-nots.

Money, of course, buys power and influence, so another factor which overlaps with material wealth is social status. Numerous studies over the past 30 years have confirmed that social status affects both physical and mental health. The Whitehall study of civil servants, for example, has been in progress since 1967. It has shown that low job status is related to higher risks of heart disease, some cancers, chronic lung disease, gastrointestinal disease, back pain, depression, suicide, sickness absence from work and self-reported ill health (Bosma *et al*, 1997). This link holds up even when the influence of lifestyle differences is accounted for. A crucial factor seems to be the degree of agency an individual enjoys at work. Those in low-status jobs who feel they have little control over their working lives are more likely to suffer from poor health. Thus, an important element of the effects of inequality appears to be not just differences in wealth, but differences in social identity, power and control over one's life.

Social divisions

A consequence of inequality is the increase in social divisions in society. One explanation for the link between inequality and poor health outcomes is the social gulf that tends to exist between people in different socio-economic groups. In the 2009 BBC Reith lectures on citizenship, Michael Sandel, Harvard Professor of Government, addressed this issue in the final lecture. Part of the problem is that we tend to talk about inequality as if the problem were how to redistribute access to private consumption. But the real problem with inequality lies in the damage it does to the civic project, to the common good:

Here's why. Too great a gap between rich and poor undermines the solidarity that democratic citizenship requires. As inequality deepens, rich and poor live increasingly separate lives. The affluent send their children to private schools in wealthy suburbs, leaving urban public schools to the children who have no alternative. A similar trend leads to the withdrawal by the privileged from other public institutions and facilities. Private health clubs replace municipal recreation centres and swimming pools. Affluent residential communities hire private security guards and rely less on public police protection. A second or third car removes the need to rely on public transportation. And so on. (Sandel, 2009)

Sandel describes how large material differences can *hollow out the public realm*, diminish what we think of as common space and damage our social relations. The trend is to spend our leisure time with people from similar socioeconomic groups – 'people like us'. Meanwhile, people from other social groups become less familiar and we find it increasingly hard to put ourselves in their shoes. Mistrust grows and easily escalates to fear and prejudice. There is increasing concentration of poverty in neglected neighbourhoods, whether it be inner-city Baltimore or a 'sink' estate in Leicester. In these areas, poor people have to cope, not only with their own poverty, but with the consequences of the deprivation of their neighbours. With greater inequality, people are more frightened of losing what they have and there is more pressure to fend for themselves and see other people as a threat. Social barriers are erected and tensions break out on the edges between different social groups. People at the bottom feel stuck and powerless – with good reason, as the relationship between income inequality and low intergenerational social mobility is strong (Blanden *et al*, 2005). Intergenerational social mobility in the UK and the USA from the 1980s onwards (perhaps surprisingly, given the mythology of the 'American dream') has been much lower than in Canada and the Scandinavian countries, where there is greater equality. This links to educational opportunities, where the picture confirms Sandel's sense that in societies where the better off are encouraged to opt out of public provision, lives are set on parallel trajectories that tend not to cross.

Such separation leads to less mutuality in relationships across social divisions and less caring about one another. Indeed, social groups become more suspicious and frightened of each other, more competitive with each other and exhibit various manifestations of envy, and defences against it, such as hostility. Kinship – the recognition of likeness and interrelatedness, and the subsequent impetus to generosity – at this societal level is severely undermined.

In a modern, relatively affluent, consumerist society, then, income inequality is a toxic influence on individuals across the social and socio-economic spectrum, and on the structure of and relationships in society: it is bad for everybody's health. Inequality, through the mechanisms explored thus far, also has a direct and negative influence on another key aspect of society: the quality and degree of *social capital*.

Social capital and health

It has been established for many years that having friends is good for you and even increases your life expectancy. Harvard Professor of Public Policy and author of *Bowling Alone: The Collapse and Revival of American Community*, Robert Putnam, claims that 'Joining and participating in just one group cuts in half your odds of dying next year!' (see http://www.bowlingalone.com).

There is also evidence that people in rich countries have fewer friends than in the past. To quote Putnam again, 'People watch *Friends* on TV – they don't have them!' (Putnam, 2000, p. 108). The extent and quality of relations between people are essential to our social fabric and as such have become a major focus of study. This is what social scientists refer to as social capital – the range and quality of positive connections between individuals and the social networks that embody people's involvement in community life.

In the 1990s, epidemiologists did a comparative study looking at death rates across states in the USA using data from the General Social Surveys and counted how many people from each state were members of voluntary organisations such as church groups and unions. In short, the higher the group membership within a state, the lower was the death rate. This held true for all causes combined, as well as deaths from coronary heart disease, cancers and infant deaths. Along the same lines, Putnam looked at social capital in the different states in relation to an index of health that included such factors as percentage of babies categorised as low birth weight, the number of people with AIDS and cancer, and death rates from different causes. He found a close link between high levels of social capital and high scores (reflecting good health) on the index. States such as Minnesota and Vermont scored high on both accounts, while states such as Louisiana and Nevada scored badly. There was also a positive correlation between social capital and measures of healthcare such as expenditure on health, numbers of hospital beds, immunisation rates and percentage of mothers receiving antenatal care (Kawachi *et al*, 1997). Perhaps unsurprisingly, people who are strongly linked together invest more in caring for each other's health.

In *Bowling Alone*, Putnam shows how Americans have become increasingly disconnected from one another and how social structures have disintegrated, impoverishing the lives of both individuals and communities. He describes three main areas of social change over the past 30 years in the USA: first, a reduction in political and civic engagement; second, a reduction in informal social ties; and third, a reduction in trust of each other. Using comparative studies of different communities with different levels of social engagement, he argues that stronger social capital (the sum total of people's involvement in community life) is linked to better health and other positive social outcomes.

Social capital, with its implication of connectedness and civic engagement, can be seen as a measure of a society's success in expressing kinship and kindness. Social capital knits society together and affects the quality of public life. It is based on and contributes to a sense of trust and reciprocity. It is also linked to equality, in a relationship that is mutually reinforcing.

Social capital can be measured using *social network analysis*, a complex methodology for exploring the relationships between people. By asking study participants to list the people they know, and which acquaintances know each other, researchers seek to represent visually and quantitatively the web of relationships around and among people. Research in a number of academic fields, including sociology, community psychology and public health, has shown that social networks operate on many levels, from families up to the level of nations. They play a critical role in determining the ways in which problems are solved and organisations are run, in addition to their effect on the health and well-being of individuals.

Social networks consist of two elements: individuals (nodes) and the relationships (social ties) between them. Once all the nodes and ties are known, one can draw pictures of the network and discern every person's position within it. Within a network, researchers analyse *clustering* and the *distance* between two people (also known as the *degree of separation*). Obesity, smoking behaviour and happiness (Christakis & Fowler, 2007, 2008; Fowler & Christakis, 2009) have all been shown to cluster; and the association holds up to three degrees removed in the social network – so, for example, one is more likely to smoke if one's friends' friends' friends smoke. Networks of the right kind, though, are also powerful positive forces.

Happiness, health and kindness

Fowler and Christakis' research on the spread of happiness is pertinent to kindness. Their data suggest that people at the core of their local networks seem more likely to be happy, while those on the periphery seem more likely to be unhappy. The authors discount the influence of similar socioeconomic status on the clustering of happy people: next-door neighbours had a much stronger influence than neighbours who lived a few doors away and who consequently had similar housing, wealth and environmental exposures. Moreover, the geographical distribution of happiness in the study was not systematically related to local levels of either income or education. In short, happiness spreads from person to person and is influenced particularly by first-degree relatives, close friends, neighbours and co-workers. The authors suggest:

Happiness is not merely a function of individual experience or individual choice but is also a property of groups of people. Indeed changes in individual happiness can ripple through social networks and generate large scale structure in the network, giving rise to clusters of happy and unhappy individuals. (Fowler & Christakis, 2009, p. 338)

Happiness is not everything and it is worth pointing out that one can be unhappy and still be a valued friend and productive citizen. Happiness does, however, have a positive effect on physical health and is increasingly being used as a measure of the overall quality of human lives, rather than economic measures such as GDP (Layard, 2005). Moreover, there is evidence that people who care about the happiness of others and the relief of misery will themselves be happier. In other words, happiness is in dynamic relation to how we treat each other – it is promoted through offering and receiving kindness.

Political implications

Mental and physical health are, then, highly influenced by levels of absolute poverty, by inequality and stress, and by the quality and closeness of the connections in society. Societies and communities that embody kinship to the extent that there is common purpose, active recognition of interdependence and responsibility for each other, equality and warm, positive interpersonal and group bonds are, very simply, healthier. These societies are overcoming the fear and anxiety involved in recognising and expressing collective kinship – and the social forces working against it. More importantly, they realise that it pays to be kind – and are willing to invest in it, emotionally, practically and financially.

If improved health is your goal, then, it is pretty clear what you must do. Policies across government departments must be directed towards:

- eradicating poverty
- energetically reducing income inequality
- promoting common identity and purpose
- communicating the value of, and supporting, combined effort and shared risk
- reducing isolation and social divisions
- supporting positive connections between people.

This is a politics of kinship and kindness. Clearly, health promotion and care will make a difference, but, whether people pay for their healthcare through taxes, private insurance or in cash, they will get poorer outcomes and value, the less these wider social and economic factors are collectively addressed. Currently, UK politics fails to take this integrated radical approach. Reduced income inequality and reinforcement of strong social capital correlate with lower drug misuse, crime, illness and family breakdown. However, society continues to address these symptoms with a complex and disconnected mixture of legal, remedial and financial weapons, rather than positively and vigorously addressing their underlying causes.

The extent of the failure in the UK to address inequality and to build social connectedness can be seen in research published in early 2010 by the National Equality Panel (NEP) (Hills, 2010) and National Centre for Social Research (NCSR) (2010). The NEP research shows that the divide between rich and poor in the UK is greater than at any time since the Second World War, and among the highest in the world. Social mobility is low, whether measured by income or profession. But the problem is deeper: it begins in the underlying public commitment to collective national life – to kinship in action. In the British Social Attitudes Survey the NCSR reports the public commitment to collective investment in the common good as being lower than it has been for many years, and the decline has been severe in recent years. Only 56% of the general public believe there is an obligation to vote (68% in 1991). Only 38% feel that government should strive to create a more equal society (51% in 1994). The number who support increased taxation to fund health, education and social services (38%) is the lowest since 1983. Although this is mitigated by a small rise in those believing that tax should stay the same, the number who feel it should fall is at its highest for over 20 years (8% in 2005, with an average over the preceding 20 years of 5%, and a steep rise since 2001).

The survey suggests that there is still a clear majority in support of pooling resources and responsibility in public services, but the degree of drift away from such commitment recently suggests real vulnerability in that social contract. Lower commitment to communal life through voting, lower understanding of interdependence, especially relating to the effects of inequality, and the signs of falling public readiness to pool resources through taxation are all signs of this vulnerability. They suggest an accelerating trend towards social fragmentation and increased inequality. A failure to restore confidence, to re-engage the public in the politics of kinship and communality, is likely to have far-reaching consequences for the health of the nation.

Successive governments have failed to embrace a genuinely integrated politics of kinship – either philosophically or in how their vision is implemented. The Labour governments from 1997 to 2010 were ideologically committed to reducing social exclusion, and espoused many ideas relating to strengthening communities and the redistribution of wealth. But inequality rose and social fragmentation appears to have increased in many ways, if the findings of the NCSR and many other reports are to be trusted. The 2010 Conservative–Liberal coalition government introduced the idea of the 'Big Society', which advocates increased voluntarism and philanthropy, public services reform – promoting voluntary, private and social enterprise – and community empowerment. This three-point strategy clearly proposes increased connectedness and involvement across society, but it has profound weaknesses if improved health and well-being are desired. Behind the laudable wish to remove bureaucracy and waste and to generate innovation, diversity and responsiveness is a clear antipathy to and denigration of large-scale state-run services. There are many things that could change for the better in publicly run services, but uncritically taking them away risks fragmentation, inconsistency, diluted expertise and lack of coordination. The 'freed' professionals risk the absence of a properly supportive infrastructure and the fracture of the working arrangements and relationships that make their work effective. Removing unnecessary bureaucracy and waste is not the same as removing vital systems that ensure that the needs of the many and of the few are addressed. Encouraging a multitude of innovative projects and organisations, whatever its merits, is not the same as ensuring a comprehensive system of services.

The idea of empowering communities is welcome, but the problems of how to promote capacity and capability, and how to resource and support an increasingly atomised public sphere *for the good of all* appear, so far, to have been neglected. The Big Society's vision of social commitment and anthropy may promote many highly valuable social initiatives but it is wider picture that is of concern. It neglects the fact that society faces ge-scale, collective problems that require systematic and comprehensive .tention, and the expert deployment of resources, well beyond the capacity and influence of individuals and local groups. Dislike of the manifold weaknesses of the 'big state' does not, in itself, prove that there is any other vehicle than the state (at a national, regional or local level) able to address these challenges.

This policy is being advanced at a time of huge reductions in public spending. Such budget reductions affect the whole system – and inevitably threaten social capital and services from whatever sector. In 2010, the UK Office for Budget Responsibility indicated that up to 500000 job losses in the public sector will occur. The 'purchasing power' of local government will be severely restricted, and this will directly affect other sectors. The Charity Commission warned in October 2010 that up to £5 billion of funding to charities could be withdrawn. Chairwoman Dame Suzi Leather said:

If you cut the charities you are cutting our ability to help each other, you are cutting what structures our neighbourliness. That is what the Big Society is all about, so you are pulling the rug out from under it. (Leather, 2010)

Underlying these risks to social capital is the reality, spelt out by the Institute for Fiscal Studies (Browne & Levell, 2010) and many others, that the poor look likely to bear a disproportionate burden of the cuts to the public sector. Inequality, then, continues.

It is hard to see how attempting to create the 'Big Society' with such limited resources and enormous challenges can come near to making up for the social costs involved in destroying the 'big state', whatever fragmented and partial opportunities for alternatives exist. The poor and vulnerable will suffer most, but all of society faces the cost of the disruption and destruction of vital services that have taken years to develop.

The crucial issues of gaining support for equality, and investment through taxes, need framing in the ethic and the vital impulse of kinship. Nowhere is there the clear, unembarrassed, assertion that sharing resources more equally and paying taxes for health, education and social services are good things, and that we all benefit enormously from doing so. Instead, income inequality has been at best tentatively discussed, and the anxiety to reassure voters that taxation will be proportionate has all but silenced any voice actively promoting the ethical argument for and collective benefits of paying taxes. To reassure the people that taxation will be fair and manageable is only good sense. But it is close to tragic to fail to communicate its value, to fail to engage the public in the vision for the good society, and to fail to argue positively for pooling resources and efforts to achieve it. The British people are inexorably falling for the idea that 'the state' is something different from the community – that 'they' take our money away from us, rather than organise valuable things to meet our needs. As important as the rational perspective is the emotional. At the heart of the resistance to unashamed promotion of equality and collective investment, it appears, is a fundamental failure to reconcile the risks of binding ourselves together with the need for, and benefits of, our doing so.

The politics of ambivalence

The 2009 US presidential election was interesting in this respect, in that Barack Obama appeared to appeal directly and powerfully to the collective kinship of the American people. Domestically, he communicated a vision of black and white, of rich and poor, of city dwellers and country people being of equal value and of a nation with rifts and divisions healed. He also stressed that success in addressing problems depended on the commitment, generosity and ingenuity of all. Internationally, he communicated a recognition of common interest, of talking, of working together to solve problems, of sharing resources and resourcefulness.

It was striking how deeply this message initially entered the American public mind – and how much it found a resonance in their hearts. Vox pop interviews following his election demonstrated how many people in the USA had heard his three-word election slogan 'Yes we can' as embodying three principles in interplay: 'yes' = positive attitude and commitment, 'we' = collective interdependency and effort, and 'can' = resourcefulness and capability. In differing languages, they showed they understood this and valued it. Strikingly, this understanding had enormous reach into the US public – it was evident among the poor and the young as much as with the better off and older adults. Indeed, the simple equation sketched above was directly expressed in a radio interview with a young, poor black woman involved in an urban welfare project.

It is no coincidence that Obama's vision had, close to its heart, healthcare reform. He expressed his inclusive and interdependent vision and his appeal to the generosity of spirit of the people most explicitly in his healthcare policy. The resistance to this reform he encountered in the USA seems to have been an expression of a mixture of the fear of interdependency and kinship and the mistaken belief that unrestrained competitive individualism is good for the citizen and for society. On the right in US politics in particular, there is a strong narrative generated by that fear and mistake – by the split between individualism and kinship. In that narrative individual liberty and well-being are mortally threatened by state-sponsored communality, by sharing risk and limits to resources. This view proposes that the good of the individual lies in facing his (for this is a very male doctrine at heart) and his close kin's circumstances alone, in buying assistance for difficulties with his own hard-earned cash, in a creative struggle to overcome hardship and rise. A cherished idea in the American dream – the land of opportunity – is challenged by the evidence on social mobility and health. Nonetheless, the right's fixation with individualism and the 'privatised family' endures.

There is, of course, much to be admired and valued in the optimism and vigour of US individualism. It is not the pluralist, the courageous, the creative aspects of US culture that need questioning. It is the phobic, even hysterical, reaction to interdependency and communality that raises concern. The evidence says that hitching our wagons together, mutual support, curbing our own desires in favour of equality and investing our resources in our common destiny improves everyone's lot. The American right says no. The liberty to choose to buy healthcare – as much or as expensive as the individual can afford – is paramount.

The political drama over healthcare in the USA can be seen, then, as a struggle between two responses to the value and danger of kinship. Obama was publicly asserting the value of kinship at a whole-community level and advocating the generous sharing of risks and resources. The political right asserted the necessity of freedom from the restrictions and compromises of such interdependence. This struggle represents the split between individualism and kinship noted before, and seems to be fuelled by the threatening nature of kindness.

Obama's falling public ratings in 2010 seemed to reflect a movement in which the American people have swung between these poles. They appeared to have retreated from being profoundly moved and inspired by his appeal to kinship and kindness, to a *loss of nerve* in the enterprise similar to what may be happening in the UK in relation to the NHS. This loss of nerve may reflect just how threatening kinship is. The understandable anxieties aroused by collectively facing the nation's problems appear to have been a fertile ground for sowing doubt and asserting individualism – even for suggesting that Obama's appeal to solidarity and kinship was actively evil.

Obama's vision and invitation were supported by the evidence. The emergence of strong voices to champion a similar vision in the UK is urgent in the light of the drift away from it. But the lesson from the USA is not just that offering such a vision is possible, but that we must understand and address the profound *ambivalence* we have towards kinship and kindness if it is to be sustained. It is interesting in this respect that Wilkinson & Pickett's book has triggered a volley of criticism, with pieces appearing under emotive titles such as 'Beware false prophets' (Saunders, 2010) and 'The spirit level delusion' (Snowdon, 2010), despite accumulating evidence from meta-analyses in peer-reviewed journals (Kondo *et al*, 2009). Given the controversy it has attracted, Professor Michael Sargent of the National Institute for Medical Research, London, writing in *Nature*, felt the need to reassure readers that 'the statistics are from reputable independent sources' (Sargent, 2010). But there is the danger that mud sticks. These vehement and ideological attacks may undermine confidence in a strongly argued case for equality. Whatever the technical debates about the use and presentation of statistics, it is clear that the politics of equality and kinship, the idea that the country would be a better place for us all if we were less divided, attracts highly anxious opposition and denigration.

Why should the creative vitality of independence and individuality have to be defined *against* kinship and collective kindness? How can we keep our nerve and trust that they can be realised together? In the next chapter, the meaning and place of kindness in the delivery of healthcare is explored, and the case made for it being valued and understood as a very powerful force for improvement and efficiency.

References

Blanden, J., Gregg, P. & Machin, S. (2005) *Intergenerational Mobility in Europe and North America*. Centre for Economic Performance, London School of Economics.

BMJ (1996) The big idea (Editor's choice). *BMJ*, **312**, 20 April (http://www.bmj.com/content/312/7037/0.full).

Bosma, H., Marmot, M. G., Hemingway, H., *et al* (1997) Low job control and risk of coronary heart disease in Whitehall II (prospective cohort) study. *BMJ*, **314**, 558–565.

Browne, J. & Levell, P. (2010) *The Distributional Effect of Tax and Benefit Reforms to be Introduced Between June 2010 and April 2014: A Revised Assessment*. Institute for Fiscal Studies.

Christakis, N. A. & Fowler, J. H. (2007) The spread of obesity in a large social network over 32 years. *New England Journal of Medicine*, **357**, 370–379.

Christakis, N. A. & Fowler, J. H. (2008) The collective dynamics of smoking in a large social network over 32 years. *New England Journal of Medicine*, **358**, 2249–2258.

Commission on Social Determinants of Health (2008) *Closing the Gap in a Generation: Health Equity Through Action on the Social Determinants of Health*. World Health Organization. Available at http://www.who.int/social_determinants/thecommission/finalreport/en/index.html (last accessed March 2011).

Department of Health (2000) *The National Health Service Plan*. HMSO.

Department of Health (2009) *Tackling Health Inequalities: 10 Years On*. HMSO.

Fowler, J. H. & Christakis, N. A. (2009) Dynamic spread of happiness in a large social network: longitudinal study of the Framingham Heart Study social network. *BMJ*, **338**, 23–27.

Hertzman, C., Siddiqi, A. A., Hertzman, E., *et al* (2010) Tackling inequality: get them while they're young. *BMJ*, **340**, 346–348.

Hills, J. (2010) *An Anatomy of Economic Inequality in the UK*. National Equality Panel Report. HMSO.

Kawachi, I., Kennedy, B. P., Lochner, K., *et al* (1997) Social capital, income inequality, and mortality. *American Journal of Public Health*, **87**, 1491–1498.

Kondo, N., Sembajwe, G., Kawachi, I., *et al* (2009) Income inequality, mortality and self rated health: meta-analysis of multilevel studies. *BMJ*, **339**, b4471.

Layard, R. (2005) *Happiness: Lessons From a New Science*. Penguin.

Leather, S. (2010) Spending review: cuts could cost charities 'billions'. *Politics Show*, 24 October, BBC1.

Marmot, M. (2010) *Fair Society, Healthy Lives*. The Marmor Review (http://www.marmotreview.org/AssetLibrary/pdfs/Reports/FairSocietyHealthyLives.pdf).

National Centre for Social Research (2010) *British Social Attitudes Survey 2010*. HMSO.

Pickett, K. E. & Wilkinson, R. (2009) Greater equality and better health. *BMJ*, **339**, b4320.

Putnam, R. D. (2000) *Bowling Alone: The Collapse and Revival of American Community*. Simon and Schuster Paperbacks.

Sandel, M. (2009) Reith lectures 2009, lecture 4: 'Politics of the Common Good', broadcast 30 June, Radio 4.

Sargent, M. (2010) Why inequality is fatal. *Nature*, **458**, 1109–1110.

Saunders, P. (2010) Beware false prophets. *Policy Exchange*, 8 July.

Schwartz, B.(2004) *The Paradox of Choice: Why More is Less*. HarperCollins.

Snowdon, C. (2010) *The Spirit Level Delusion: Fast-Checking the Left's New Theory on Everything*. Democracy Institute/Little Dice.

Subramanian, S. V. & Kawachi, I. (2004) Income inequality and health: what we have learned so far? *Epidemiologic Review*, **26**, 78–91.

Walberg, P, McKee, M., Shkolnikov, V., *et al* (1998) Economic change, crime and mortality crisis in Russia: regional analysis. *BMJ*, **317**, 312–318.

Wilkinson, R. G. (1996) *Unhealthy Societies: The Affliction of Inequality*. Routledge.

Wilkinson, R. G. & Pickett, K. (2009) *The Spirit Level. Why More Equal Societies Almost Always Do Better*. Allen Lane (Penguin).

CHAPTER 3

Building the case for kindness

Ability is what you're capable of doing.
Motivation determines what you do.
Attitude determines how well you do it.
(Variously attributed to Raymond Chandler and Lou Holtz)

Most of us would agree with the proposition that kindness promotes a sense of well-being. But does it make a real difference? Is there evidence for a link between kindness and health, the idea that kindness can be therapeutic and directly improve satisfaction, treatment and outcomes? This chapter explores this idea as well as its corollary – that a lack of kindness can be anti-therapeutic and degrade the delivery of healthcare and its outcomes. The discussion refers to a selection of subjective narratives from individuals as well as information from surveys and data about satisfaction and complaints. It draws on more objective data linking measurable physical improvement with aspects of kind care, and what is going on in the brain when someone is giving or receiving kindness.

The patient experience

There is a clear link between kindness and patient satisfaction. Stories from patients and their carers illustrate again and again that kindness, or its absence, touches them deeply, colours their experience of being a patient and is often what they remember years afterwards. The following is from an article in the *BMJ* written by a general practitioner:

Friends and relatives who have been inpatients recently all have similar complaints – never seeing a nurse except when drugs were being handed out, no-one offering reassurance or information, days going by without any contact with senior medical staff, virtually having to beg for help moving up the bed or getting to the toilet, repeated requests for analgesia. Two elderly relatives developed pressure sores after straightforward surgery, and one lost six per cent of her body weight after a joint replacement because of prolonged nausea that was inadequately managed. It's these experiences, and not the skilful surgery, that patients remember and tell their friends about. And it's these that make patients, especially elderly patients, dread being in hospital. (Teale, 2007)

This description reflects many aspects of our own experience with family and friends who have been ill. Of course, one or two would not be alive without the advances that have taken place in medicine over the past 10–20 years; and others are enjoying a quality of life much enhanced by modern drugs, cataract removal and joint replacement. But there has been much misery and anxiety caused by some aspects of their care in hospital, such as being moved from ward to ward without explanation, unsympathetic communication, inadequate pain relief and sleepless nights as a result of other patients whose attempts to attract the attention of the nurses are unheard. One of our relatives still feels angry about the callous way he was handed (without warning) a bag of soiled clothing to wash as his wife lay dying. Another had a rare type of Guillain–Barré syndrome and, while she was impressively diagnosed and pulled through the crisis, her difficulty feeding was ignored and no special diet was provided, despite her extreme difficulty swallowing. Another was tormented by a very itchy rash, easily treated but neglected for days. It is hard to imagine these situations occurring if there had been more kindness – and the attentiveness and understanding it nourishes – within the system.

Many people's stories about their experience of healthcare centre around the degree and quality of kindness they have (or have not) experienced. Often these accounts are complaints about the absence of kindness, the sheer thoughtlessness, lack of care and inhumanity in the system. Sometimes they describe the power of small – but highly relevant – acts of kindness to transform an otherwise miserable experience of suffering. Most often they are a mixture of the two.

In addition to direct anecdotal feedback from people we know who have recently been patients, the patient opinion website (http://www.patientopinion.org.uk) has been helpful in offering a wider variety of perspectives. A sample of letters posted on the website during the week we were writing this chapter yielded the following:

The care given to my husband who suffered from a brain tumour during his stay was amazing. The care given by nurses and doctors was way above the call of duty. They showed such kindness and helped him preserve his dignity in a difficult situation. (Head 563)

I hardly remember much about the actual attack as I was at the time too stressed about why this bloody heartburn had started to join up with my left arm in a battle to convince my chest that there was an elephant sitting on my ribs – And that is all I can remember about that day really, except all the kindness, consideration and warmth. I felt I was being looked after by some of the best in Britain. (DMF)

My mother unfortunately suffered a major stroke whilst she was staying with us. From arriving at A&E, the care that my mother received and the kindness shown to us as her family, was tremendous. All staff, although very busy, kept us fully informed from the outset with regard to her condition. I would like to ensure that the PCT are aware of our gratitude and appreciation to all of the staff we encountered – including the ladies who delivered the drinks and meals and those who keep the ward scrupulously clean. (Grail 716)

I attended in May and August for a double hip replacement. The best thing about my treatment was the kindness – My first stay in May made a frightening situation into an organised and calm experience. (Elated 866)

Clearly, there is no claim to this being a representative sample but it does seem that most of the positive opinions mention the word kindness and often link this with other key aspects of good practice.

Information from patient satisfaction surveys and data from official complaints (Patients Association, 2008, 2010) show a remarkable degree of overlap with the more negative opinions posted on the patient opinion website. All confirm how deeply troubled people are when their basic physical needs are not met. There are a worrying number of accounts of patients being left in soiled bedding and clothing, and of personal hygiene and nutritional needs being neglected. Respect for patients' dignity is fundamental to a kind approach to care. A number of complaints focus on bedside curtains or room doors being left open when patients are receiving intimate care; and clothing being inappropriate – particularly gowns failing adequately to protect modesty.

All such complaints no doubt reflect major systemic problems, but they are mediated through individual members of staff, who have the opportunity to transform the experience for the patient. It may, for example, be necessary for a service to postpone a general practice or out-patient appointment at short notice (another common focus of complaints) but a kind call from someone explaining the reasons and apologising, can, at least, prevent the patient feeling overlooked, uncared for and neglected. Anyone who has ever waited anxiously for a medical consultation knows how slowly time passes and how difficult it is to think of anything else or get on with one's life in the interim. Likewise, in modern highly specialised hospitals, it may not be possible to avoid moving a patient from ward to ward and from one highly technical investigation to the next, but a sense of continuity, even just the words of a kind, sensitive, reassuring porter who treats the patient like a person, not a parcel, can make a huge difference. One of the problems here is that events that are uniquely personal and profoundly significant to the patient are part of the day-to-day routine for clinical and administrative staff. Patients often comment on how they were made to feel a nuisance.

Crowding out the human

A very simple, but telling, illustration of the tension between patients' felt experience and an impersonal system is made by Giskin Day and Naomi

Carter in 'Wards of the roses' (Day & Carter, 2009). They note the trend in both individual wards and entire hospitals to prohibit flowers. Reasons given include avoiding the depletion of oxygen in the air, avoiding water spillage over electrical equipment and the risk of infection. Apart from the sheer nonsense of the oxygen argument, none of these justifications has a secure base in evidence. Although flower water, not surprisingly, contains bacteria, rigorous studies have emphatically concluded that bedside flowers pose no threat to health (Cohn, 2009). What is interesting is just how widespread the prohibition is, despite this evidence. More mundane – and perhaps more honest – reasons given by nurses and managers are the inconvenience of changing water regularly and the problems involved in disposing of dead flowers.

Here is a matter that is important to patients and their visitors, which is, apparently, inconsequential in modern healthcare delivery. Even if we can see emerging social trends that value other such tokens, it should be remembered that the majority of people in UK acute hospital care are aged over 65. The gift of flowers is a ritual valued across the world: it reinforces meaningful relationships, expressing concern, love and friendship. Such gifts are particularly important to patients in hospital, because they demonstrate social ties beyond visiting hours and mark out a small, personalised space. Cohn uses this instance to illustrate a wider issue. Efficiency is split off from and set against the quality of patient experience:

The decision to ban flowers ... is not the articulation of rational science but increased rationalisation, in the sociological sense, which equates with technological efficiency coupled with greater bureaucracy and accountability. (Cohn, 2009, p. 1389)

The processes of routinisation and institutionalisation often undermine kindness. But the fact that situations where small acts of kindness can make a difference are routine can also be seen as an opportunity. On the whole, patients realise that today's healthcare staff are desperately pushed for time, but really appreciate a kindly exchange while the doctor re-sites an intravenous needle or the nurse changes the infusion bag. Routine tasks such as taking blood pressure, helping a patient sit up or emptying a catheter bag can be done mechanically or in a way that conveys sensitivity, gentleness and respect. The more intimate and personal the task, the more these qualities are appreciated. There are tasks such as bathing an elderly person that offer extended opportunity to build a relationship and get to know the person in the patient; and other situations where this can be conveyed with a kind smile or a reassuring hand on a shoulder.

All the evidence from patients themselves is that they *want to be seen and known* as the people they are, not just as a list of problems. In among the complaints and squalid detail of poor practice, the encouraging message in patients' narratives is that ordinary kind behaviour is really appreciated. Something as seemingly small as making the effort to pronounce a name properly or helping to fit a hearing aid can make a huge difference to a patient's experience and sense of well-being. The simple story below demonstrates this difference. The storyteller, Jane, is a thoughtful woman who recently faced over a year of treatment for cancer, including radical, high-risk surgery. It is the link between the tiny gesture she remembers and the effects on her relationship with her doctor that speaks volumes:

The consultant who has been treating me does not fit my stereotype of the cold, distant, arrogant surgeon at all. After any examination, he always offers me a hand to help me get up from the examination table. This small gesture of kindness I have found very significant. It has helped me feel able to communicate with him in an open and honest way as a person, not just another ill patient.

Seeing the person in the patient

The heading above is taken from a review paper by the King's Fund that launched its 'Point of Care' programme, which aims to improve patients' experience of care in hospital and to 'help staff deliver the sort of care they would like for themselves and their own families' (Goodrich & Cornwell, 2008). The project is an example of some of the work in train to translate concepts such as personalisation and person-centred care into real change in hospital practice. This aim resonates with definitions of kindness that focus on the shared root with *kinship* and *kindred* (see Chapter 1). Kind staff have a sense of shared humanity and see in the patient someone who is part of the flow of life and essentially the same as themselves.

The simply stated aim also conveys an important element of kindness that comes up frequently in patient narratives, namely that kind behaviour is usually about very ordinary, day-to-day things such as speaking clearly when someone's a bit deaf, remembering someone's special diet, taking the time to help someone brush their hair or bothering to clean someone's spectacles. One of the commonest complaints made by hospital patients is that call bells are left out of reach: surely something that a bit more caring attentiveness could easily remedy and something that should naturally follow from empathising with the sense of powerlessness experienced by people in a state of vulnerability.

But if it is that easy, why does it not happen more often? What would break through the hazards of workload, stress and routine and bring about such behaviour? It is good to see words like *compassion* appearing in recent health policy and in initiatives like the King's Fund project. In the current climate, however, there is a danger of the development of yet more standards, specifications and procedures to promote such behaviour. This process is unlikely to reap the benefits hoped for unless ways of promoting and supporting *attentive kindness in everyday practice* are brought to bear on the daily lives of staff.

The link with *attentiveness* is important: it is hard to act kindly if one is inattentive and – turning it round the other way – kindness promotes and focuses attentiveness. Kindness at once derives from and prompts a combination of vigilant observation, active listening and the art of holding the patients' needs in mind.

It would appear, then, that kindness, communicating fellow feeling and warmth, attentiveness to patients as people, and expressed through actions attuned to their suffering and needs, is strongly associated with patient satisfaction. The theory and research, however, go further: they suggest strong links between kindness and effective care and, consequently, *outcomes*.

The importance of a good therapeutic alliance

We can see how much patients value being treated kindly and that the foundation of kindness lies in the capacity to empathise with patients and their vulnerability, and to see beyond the manifestations of illness to the person inside. Staff who work in teams where such an attitude is encouraged are much less likely to allow their patients to suffer through lack of attentiveness, sensitivity and respect. It is well to remember, however, that a therapeutic relationship involves two people. Patients are not just passive recipients of care. They bring their strengths, foibles, fears and particular personality characteristics. Most important in this context is their capacity for trust.

Our sense of well-being is very much influenced by how much we are able to put our trust in other people. This is most obvious when we are ill and vulnerable and highly dependent on the care of others. Most of us experience some anxiety when we – sometimes literally – have to put ourselves in someone else's hands, hopefully informed, but sometimes blindly. For some, the degree of anxiety can be crippling: not only will it cause misery in itself, but it may detrimentally affect communication, reduce compliance with treatment and undermine the capacity for healing. People who are anxious and mistrustful are less able to think about themselves, to share information with clinical staff, or to commit themselves actively to treatment and associated lifestyle changes.

The *therapeutic alliance* is a term commonly used in psychotherapy and counselling; it describes the quality and strength of the relationship between the therapist and client. It links to the concept of trust, which in any relationship is affected by the baggage each party brings in terms of experiences from the past, as well as what happens in the here and now. A good therapeutic alliance is a relationship where the patient believes that the therapist has the patient's best interest at heart and that their interest in the patient is benign. Over 4000 papers and dissertations have been written on this subject over the past 30 years and more than 24 different scales developed to measure it. While the degree to which the therapeutic alliance contributes to the variance in outcome is debated, there is consistent evidence and agreement that a good outcome is more likely where a good therapeutic alliance has been established (Cooper, 2008).

Certain qualities and behaviours in the therapist will foster a strong therapeutic alliance. These include warmth, friendliness, genuineness, openness (as in wisely judged self-disclosure), empathy (entering the private perceptual world of the other and having an accurate, felt understanding of the person's experience) and positive regard (a warm, non-judgemental acceptance of the other and their experience). Many of these relational factors are highly correlated, with some authors suggesting that, from the clients' perspective, there is really just one main relational variable: experiencing the therapist as *caring/involved* (Williams & Chambless, 1990). The feeling of really mattering to their therapists or of service beyond normal expectations summed up in the phrase *going the extra mile* has also been identified in the research as contributing to positive outcomes (McMillan & McLeod, 2006).

The qualities that promote a good therapeutic alliance are integral to kindness. What is more, the research shows that where a strong therapeutic alliance has been established, patients tend to respond better to challenges, are less likely to drop out of treatment, and recover more quickly when the therapist is perceived as making a mistake. A similar finding has been established in group therapy. People will feel safer and therefore more able to make constructive and therapeutic use of a group setting where there is a strong sense of group cohesion, which, in turn, is fostered by the therapist modelling a transparent, inclusive, non-judgemental, accepting style of intervention (Burlingame *et al*, 2002; Minkulince *et al*, 2005). Even where self-help manuals and web-based therapeutic programmes have been shown to be efficacious with relatively specific behavioural problems such as smoking, there is evidence that some interpersonal contact seems to boost their efficacy (van Boeijen *et al*, 2005).

Research indicates that therapists can underestimate the importance of relational factors, preferring to believe their efficacy derives from their professional mastery (Feifel & Eells, 1963) when to a large extent it may come from helping to create an atmosphere of warmth and tolerance. Clients, on the other hand, consistently ascribe most importance to relational factors such as having someone care, listen and understand and provide encouragement and reassurance (Bohart & Tallman, 1999) and the therapist's calm, sympathetic listening, support and approval (Ryan & Gizynski, 1971). Interestingly, the positive correlation between the quality of the therapeutic relationship and therapeutic outcome is just as strong in non-relationally orientated therapies such as cognitive–behavioural therapy as in psychodynamic and humanistic therapies, which have always framed the therapeutic relationship as central to the therapeutic model.

Much of the work in NHS psychotherapy is with people who are highly anxious and vulnerable, with a deep-seated tendency to be mistrustful. But accident, physical illness, pain, uncertainty and admission to hospital can trigger the same combination in all of us. It seems that kindness can mitigate this by building trust, which, in turn, underpins a good therapeutic alliance. This will directly improve patients' sense of well-being, but also promotes communication and cooperation and stands patients in good stead when things are particularly difficult, for example when taking in complex information, managing bad news and recovering more quickly if things go wrong. The interplay between kindness, empathy, trust and a strong therapeutic alliance is well illustrated by Jane (who spoke of her surgeon's kindness earlier):

I have had complete trust in both the surgeon and the oncologist who have been treating me for cancer. When I have had decisions to make about the choices open to me in the next steps of treatment, each of them, while discussing the possible options, has also offered a more personal opinion. In the case of the male surgeon, what he would recommend if his wife were in this situation, and in the case of the female oncologist what she herself would do given this choice of options.

Because of the trust I have in both of them, this has made the decision about what to do next very easy for me. I have not felt the need to examine statistics, or trawl the internet for information. I have felt confident in making my decision given that my doctors, whilst being experts in their fields and having my best interests at heart, were also able and willing to empathise with me and with my situation.

There is, then, strong evidence, from research and from patient experience, that attentive kindness builds the sort of relationship between staff and patient within which reduction of suffering, increased trust, better communication, better understanding and diagnosis, and better cooperation make effective care more possible, and more likely. Interestingly, there appears to be a biological, as well as a psychological, dimension to this linkage.

The biological effects of kindness

Attachment theory is a model of caring relationships influenced by evolutionary biology, ethology and object relations psychoanalysis that shows we are biologically designed to respond positively to kindness throughout our lives. The model has given rise to a huge amount of empirical research looking at the formation of close relationships in early infancy and the transactional patterns that are set up and have a tendency to remain constant throughout life. The original proponent of attachment theory was John Bowlby, who, as a paediatrician and psychoanalyst, was interested in the effects of early parenting. This led him to pioneer a World Health Organization study looking at the physical and psychological health of the many thousands of children orphaned during the Second World War (Holmes, 1993).

Attachment behaviour in infant animals is instinctive and serves to maintain proximity to the attachment figure, thereby improving the chance of survival. In normal human development, attachment behaviour is prolonged; it forges a strong bond between infant and main caregiver(s), allowing for a lengthy period of nurtured development. Proximity seeking is at its height between the ages of 6 months and 2 years, although this period of sensitivity varies from person to person and is more flexible than first thought. Separation from the primary caregiver at this time results in anxiety and anger and, if prolonged, will lead to sadness and despair. An inaccessible or unresponsive caregiver will trigger anxious attachment behaviour in the infant and there is some evidence that the quality of attunement to the infant is more important than the amount of time spent together. Early experience with caregivers gradually gives rise to an *internal working model* of social relationships. This is a system of thoughts, memories, beliefs, expectations, emotions and behaviours about the self and others which will continue to develop throughout life, depending on experience, but which has a tendency to be heavily influenced by the patterns established during the sensitive period of infancy.

A good attachment with the caregiver will act as a *secure base* for the infant/toddler to explore the surroundings and there is a well-established relationship between the strength of the internal attachment model and a child's exploratory behaviour and willingness to stray further from the attachment figure. Research studies have explored this, observing and categorising attachment behaviour in infants (Ainsworth, 1989), as well as developing tools to analyse adult attachment styles and caregiver behaviour (Main, 1995). Threats to felt security in the infant include prolonged absence, communication breakdown, emotional unavailability, signs of rejection or abandonment, and outright hostility. This same list will continue to trigger insecurity in adult life and will lead to distress, problems with dependency and fear of change. Likewise, positive qualities in the caregiver include consistency, emotional attunement and a repertoire of soothing behaviours, including sensitive touching. Throughout life, our attachment systems will be triggered by anxiety, fear, illness, extreme tiredness and separation, and will usually respond positively to caring and kindness.

There is growing evidence that the quality of caregiving shapes the development of the neurological systems which regulate stress and self-soothing. Over the past 30 years, there has been a huge leap forward in our understanding of how the brain functions. This has confirmed not only that warm, attuned caring in early life can turn genes on and off and influence the way our brains develop (Depue & Morrone-Strupinsky, 2005) but also that throughout life the experience of kindness actually continues to nourish our brains by triggering the release of endorphins (naturally produced opiate-like substances) and oxytocin (produced in large quantities during breast-feeding and particularly responsible for the feeling of closeness) (Carter, 1998). Put very simply, neurobiologists have identified an emotion regulatory system where millions of coordinated brain cells are programmed to be activated by kind, soothing, affectionate behaviour to produce a mental state of peaceful contentment and safety.

In case there is any confusion, nurturing such a state is not the same as 'positive thinking'. The onus in 'positive thinking' is on the individual rather than the interpersonal and, when taken to extremes, can be felt as persecutory or guilt inducing. The American writer Barbara Ehrenreich, for example, in her book *Smile or Die* (2010), describes her experience of being diagnosed with breast cancer and, while expecting to discover some sort of supportive sisterhood, was surprised to encounter a tidal wave of injunctions to be positive and even grateful for the experience. Her complaints about the debilitating effects of the treatment were criticised as bad attitude and expressions of horror and dread were taboo. Despite a poor evidence base to support the claim that positive thinking affects outcome in cancer patients, it seems that many American patients experience their failure to think positively as deeply troubling (Ehrenreich, 2010). This 'positive thinking' is not the same as the sense of safety that can be nourished by kindness and that has a neurobiological basis.

The direct effect of kindness on healing

The *placebo effect* is well established in medicine: it is the phenomenon whereby patients who believe they are receiving a bona fide treatment will be more likely to report improved symptoms, even if, unbeknown to them, the supposed treatment is an inert sugar pill. Hypotheses abound as to why this might be so, but presumably the instillation of hope contributes. Certainly, it seems likely that the quality of the therapeutic relationship is a key element. This was borne out by a literature review of research on the placebo effect (Turner *et al*, 1994) which concluded that 'the quality of the interaction between physician and patient can be extremely influential in patient outcomes'.

There appear to be no studies on healthcare outcomes where kindness itself is the defined focus of exploration. Kindness is a broad, inclusive concept and may mean slightly different things to different people. But there are promising signs. In the field of mental health, there are comparative outcome studies measuring important constituents of kindness such as empathy and warmth, and associated qualities such as attunement and unconditional positive regard. Where the focus is general health, one study was able to show that patients give more useful information about their symptoms and concerns when the staff member shows empathy (Epstein *et al*, 2005) and that this leads to greater diagnostic accuracy. A number of studies make the link between high levels of anxiety and delayed healing (e.g. Cole-King & Harding, 2001; Weinman *et al*, 2008); and, as we have seen, treating people kindly can help to reduce anxiety levels. Another study compared 'compassionate care' against 'normal care' in a group of frequent attenders at an accident and emergency department and showed that patients assigned to 'compassionate care' had fewer repeat visits and were more satisfied with their care (Rendelmeir *et al*, 1995).

Generally speaking, though, there is very little research, outside the field of mental health, investigating the therapeutic effects of kindness and its associated qualities. Reasons for this include: the practical difficulties inherent in researching and measuring a concept so broad and loosely defined; the bias towards quantitative research as opposed to qualitative;

and the fact that most research funding in healthcare is sponsored by drug companies. Another reason may be our ambivalence towards the concept of kindness, the possibility that, at some level, we are more anxious about kindness than we are consciously aware.

The King's Fund Point of Care programme referred to earlier (Firth-Cozens & Cornwell, 2009) looked at compassionate care in acute hospital settings and suggests the following research agenda, which includes, or could be adapted to, the phenomenon of kindness:

- agree definitions for compassion and ways of assessing it
- agree and assess uncompassionate care (e.g. food placed too far from patients to reach; patients being moved from ward to ward; patients being prepared for procedures and operations which then do not take place)
- test whether patients know when kind words and behaviours are not supported by emotional factors, and whether this matters to them
- investigate whether increasing compassionate care promotes better clinical outcomes and patient satisfaction
- develop and test teaching and training methods
- investigate the relationships between stress reduction and caring behaviours
- explore how aspects of teamwork contribute to compassionate care, and which have the most impact.

Research of this kind can only be helpful – with the proviso raised earlier that the learning would be at risk of being applied in a 'technological' manner that misses the point, or, indeed, works against promoting kindness. There is, though, already enough evidence to sketch out a strong linkage between kindness and improved outcomes – in terms of reduction of suffering, effective treatment and recovery, well-being and patient satisfaction.

A virtuous circle

This chapter has highlighted the effectiveness of felt and expressed *kindness*, which promotes and is educated by *attentiveness*. It is possible to follow this linkage further. From attentive kindness emerges *attunement* of staff actions to the patient's felt and real experience. With the experience of such attuned actions, *anxiety is reduced and trust built*, which supports the building of an *effective therapeutic alliance*. Such an alliance promotes *better communication, understanding, diagnosis* and *cooperation*, and the result of this, combined with the underpinning direct experience of kindness by the patient, is *improved treatment outcomes, well-being and satisfaction*. This argument is expressed in diagrammatic form in Fig. 3.1.

There is an even more interesting dimension to this argument. Even on the basis of the changed relationship with patients indicated in Fig. 3.1, there is much to indicate the potential for a powerful *reinforcement effect*. Simply put, the more attentively kind staff are, the more their attunement

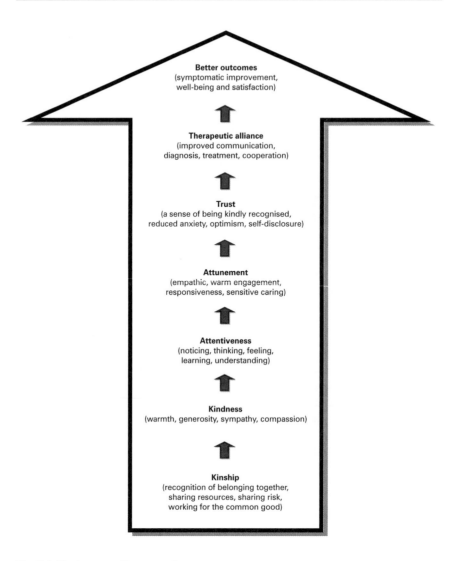

Fig. 3.1 Kindness and improved outcomes.

to the patient increases; the more that increases, the more trust is generated; the more trust, the better the therapeutic alliance; the better the alliance, the better the outcomes. The result of all this is a reduction in anxiety, improved satisfaction (for staff and patient), less defensiveness and improved conditions for kindness. The suggestion is that, as staff practise more kindly, a virtuous circle is set in motion. Our thinking in Fig. 3.1 then begins to look as if it is better expressed as a cycle, as in Fig. 3.2. In fact, the dynamics of this virtuous circle are far more complex than Fig. 3.2 suggests. It can work to bring staff and patients together to review services, and to improve them; it can be considered as a driver for improving staff morale, lowering stress

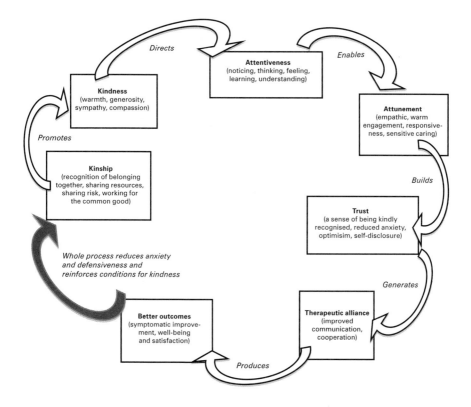

Fig. 3.2 Kindness – a virtuous circle.

levels and consequent sickness rates. Each linkage in the cycle can be seen as a 'reinforcing cycle' in itself. Kindness breeds attentiveness, which in turn inspires kindness. Similarly, a stronger therapeutic alliance does not just produce better outcomes: it also reinforces trust, which, in turn, strengthens the alliance, and so on.

These powerful dynamic processes also look as if they can contribute to *productivity* – a key challenge for all health services and, in particular for the NHS in the light of the state of public finances in the next half decade or so. A useful concept in the industrial model is that of 'getting it right first time' as a key driver for eliminating waste – of time, resources, and so on. All stages of, and the combined effect of, this cycle contribute to such effective activity. The more work is founded on kinship, motivated by kindness and expressed through attentiveness and attunement to the patient's needs, the more it is likely to be timely and 'right first time'.

Kindness rooted in kinship is a powerful concept – ethically, politically, socially and clinically – in the project of improving healthcare. It increases patient satisfaction, staff morale, clinical effectiveness and efficiency. Deep in our social and individual connection with the urge to be kind, however, lies a difficult ambivalence. Understanding that ambivalence – that human beings value and respond to kindness, but are frightened of the risks involved – is vital. At any number of levels, finding and harnessing the dynamic of our virtuous circle is hard, in the face of vicious circles that drive towards very different outcomes. It is important to understand why kindness is difficult for real, complex human individuals – citizens, patients, healthcare staff and managers.

References

Ainsworth, M. (1989) Attachments beyond infancy. *American Psychologist*, **44**, 706–716.

Bohart, A. C. & Tallman, K. (1999) *How Clients Make Therapy Work: The Process of Active Self-Healing*. American Psychological Association.

Burlingame, G. M., Fuhriman, A. & Johnson, J. E. (2002) Cohesion in group psychotherapy. In *Psychotherapy Relationships That Work: Therapist Contributions and Responsiveness to Patients* (ed. J. C. Norcross), pp. 71–87. Oxford University Press.

Carter, C. S. (1998) Neuroendocrine perspectives on social attachment and love. *Psychoneuroendocrinology*, **23**, 819–835.

Cohn, S. (2009) Where have all the flowers gone? *BMJ*, **339**, b5406.

Cole-King, A. & Harding, K. G. (2001) Psychological factors and delayed healing in chronic wounds. *Psychosomatic Medicine*, **63**, 216–220.

Cooper, M. (2008) *Essential Research Findings in Counselling and Psychotherapy*. Sage.

Day, G. & Carter, N. (2009) Wards of the roses. *BMJ*, **339**, b5257.

Depue, R. A. & Morrone-Strupinsky, J. V. (2005) A neurobehavioural model of affiliative bonding. *Behaviour and Brain Sciences*, **28**, 313–350.

Ehrenreich, B. (2010) *Smile or Die: How Positive Thinking Fooled America and the World*. Granta.

Epstein, R. M., Franks, P., Sheilds, C. G., *et al* (2005) Patient-centred communication and diagnostic testing. *Annals of Family Medicine*, **3**, 415–421.

Feifel, H. & Eells, J. (1963) Patients and therapists assess the same psychotherapy. *Journal of Consulting Psychology*, **27**, 310–318.

Firth-Cozens, J. & Cornwell, J. (2009) *The Point of Care. Enabling Compassionate Care in Acute Hospital Settings*. King's Fund.

Goodrich, J. & Cornwell, J. (2008) *Seeing the Person in the Patient*. The Point of Care Review Paper. King's Fund.

Holmes, J. (1993) *John Bowlby and Attachment Theory*. Routledge.

Main, M. (1995) Interview based adult attachment classifications: related to infant–mother and infant–father attachment. *Developmental Psychology*, **19**, 227–239.

McMillan, M. & McLeod, J. (2006) Letting go: the client's experience of relational depth. *Person-Centred and Experiential Psychotherapies*, **5**, 277–292.

Minkulince, M., Shauer, P. R., Gillath, O., *et al* (2005) Attachment, caregiving and altruism: boosting attachment security increases compassion and helping. *Journal of Personality and Social Psychology*, **89**, 817–839.

Patients Association (2008) *NHS Complaints: Who Cares? Who Can Make It Better?* Patients Association.

Patients Association (2010) *Patients Not Numbers. People Not Statistics*. Patients Association.

Rendelmeir, D. A., Molin, J. & Tibshirani, R. J. (1995) A randomised trial of compassionate care for the homeless in an emergency department. *Lancet*, **345**, 1131–1134.

Ryan, V. L. & Gizynski, M. N. (1971) Behavior therapy in retrospect – patients' feelings about their behavior therapies. *Journal of Consulting and Clinical Psychology*, **37**, 1–9.

Teale, K. (2007) What's wrong with the wards? *BMJ*, **334**, 97.

Turner, J. A., Deyo, R. A., Loeser, J. D., *et al* (1994) The importance of the placebo effects in pain treatment and research. *JAMA*, **271**, 1609–1614.

Van Boeijen, C. A., van Balkom, A., van Oppen, P., *et al* (2005) Efficacy of self-help manuals for anxiety disorders in primary care: a systematic review. *Family Practice*, **22**, 192–196.

Weinman, J., Ebrecht, M., Scott, S., *et al* (2008) Enhanced wound healing after emotional disclosure intervention. *British Journal of Health Psychology*, **13**, 95–102.

Williams, K. E. & Chambless, D. L. (1990) The relationship between therapist characteristics and outcome of in vivo exposure treatment for agoraphobia. *Behaviour Therapy*, **21**, 111–116.

Part II
The struggle with kindness

CHAPTER 4

Managing feelings of love and hate

There is nothing heavier than compassion. Not even one's own pain weighs so heavy as the pain one feels for someone [else] ... pain intensified by the imagination and prolonged by a hundred echoes. (Milan Kundera, *The Unbearable Lightness of Being*)

The pull away from kindness

Why do seemingly caring people behave unkindly? As one author put it, 'how do good staff become bad?' (Farquharson, 2004, p. 12). There are many dimensions to even a partial answer to this question. In this chapter, we look at some of the processes at work at the individual level.

First, it seems appropriate to remind or acquaint ourselves with the extreme circumstances that developed in the Mid-Staffordshire NHS Trust, in the English Midlands, between 2005 and 2009, starting with an excerpt from the executive summary of the report of the inquiry (Francis, 2010, p. 10):

Requests for assistance to use a bedpan or to get to and from the toilet were not responded to. Patients were often left on commodes or in the toilet for far too long. They were also left in sheets soaked with urine and faeces for considerable periods of time, which was especially distressing for those whose incontinence was caused by *Clostridium difficile*. Considerable suffering and embarrassment were caused to patients as a result.

There were accounts suggesting that the attitude of some nursing staff to these problems left much to be desired. Some families felt obliged or were left to take soiled sheets home to wash or to change beds when this should have been undertaken by the hospital and its staff. Some staff were dismissive of the needs of patients and their families.

Although the main focus of the recommendations following the inquiry addressed the systemic failings, the evidence given by patients and their relatives describes in grim detail some glaring indifference and cruelty on the part of individuals. Similar themes are apparent in the recent report of the Patients Association (2010). That report was the focus of an article in the *BMJ* which indicated that such problems, while varying in degree, are widespread (Jones, 2010). How do we begin to make sense of the more extreme cases of abuse and neglect? And is there any link between these extremes and the rest of us?

An important key is to understand that motivation is almost always mixed and more complex than it at first appears. The fundamental ambivalence towards kindness based on the risk it exposes people to through sharing the vulnerability and needs of others has been discussed in Chapter 1. But ambivalence is driven by other forces. Why do workers in healthcare choose the jobs they do? The profession? The specialty? The patient group? They may well offer a quick, ready, off-the-peg response, but altruism, vocation and commitment are very likely mixed with other motives relating to what they (and all of us!) seek through status, role identity and community. It might be important to look deeper, explore motivations that go all the way back to early experiences of death and illness and styles of caring – or lack of caring. Sometimes people find new light is thrown on this question many years into their careers, when they are emotionally thrown by feelings in relation to a particular patient or clinical issue that requires some introspection to sort out.

Choice of profession or of patient group often reflects personal history; for example, an individual might choose a career in intellectual disabilities because a sibling has Down syndrome, or get interested in medicine because of personal experience as a diabetic, or want to work in public health because a heavy-smoking parent died of lung cancer. Such personal links can be a driving force and source of compassion and commitment – the health service is full of such people and benefits enormously. But there is a danger, where the links are not fully conscious and understood, that this drive can tip over into the type of demanding zeal that can alienate others – patients and colleagues – and lead too easily to overwork and burnout.

The wounded healer

Psychoanalytic thinking suggests that people are driven, often without being aware, to seek ways in the present to deal with problematic or unresolved hopes, hurts and fears from the past, especially infancy and childhood. The choice of profession or of client group very often reflects and offers a theatre for people to play out wounded, unresolved, even aggressive or sadistic elements of their personalities. In these cases the unconscious motivation is often to heal a sick, or dead, family member and the guilt and fear of facing failure can become channelled into a relentless drive to work ever harder. Unfortunately, the choice of work brings not only the opportunity for reparation and healing, but also repeats the experience of failing the incurable, which, in turn, further feeds the associated emotional drive to apply oneself to this impossible task. This can become a vicious circle. Such people often make harsh, unforgiving task masters, not just to themselves but to their colleagues, and even sometimes to their patients, whom they may unconsciously blame for not responding positively to their heroic efforts. The potential for depression and burnout is obvious and this in turn can eat into the capacity for careful attention to patients, or worse, nourish resentment and mistreatment.

Many people learn through painful experience that their greatest strengths can also be weaknesses. For example, someone much loved as a charismatic teacher can also be narcissistic and greedy for attention; someone whose obsessional traits mean they have an admirable eye for detail in one area of their work may otherwise be an ultra-critical and controlling colleague. It is important to be curious about oneself, to recognise the shadow side to the declared motivation for choosing the job that one does, and to be aware of resonances between the work and life experiences. The importance of self-awareness and insight is dramatically stated in the much quoted words, 'physician, heal thyself'.

Intrinsic horrors and anxieties

The relationship with the work one does is not fixed and there is the potential for many types of experience along the way to push one to behave in an unkind manner or get stuck in an unkind state of mind. Studies confirm that the majority of healthcare students are motivated by the wish to make things better but during their training become more distanced from patients and less empathic (Lowenstein, 2008; Wear & Zarconi, 2008). Many a clinician will be conscious of something they found particularly painful and distressing and able to see how this caused them to withdraw emotionally from patients and colleagues for a while.

It is worth trying to stand back and consider the sort of things people working in healthcare actually have to do. For it is easy to forget the appalling nature of some of the jobs carried out by NHS staff day in, day out – the damage, the pain, the mess they encounter, the sheer stench of diseased human flesh and its waste products. It takes energy and concentration to be in the right state of mind so as not to physically recoil and express disgust. It is common to say that this state of mind involves 'professional detachment', but it also takes courage and 'human' kindness. The detail in the report of the Mid-Staffordshire inquiry reminds us of the shocking extremes of unkindness when failure of bodily functions are not managed sensitively and efficiently. For example, one woman told of finding her mother-in-law, a 96-year-old woman with dementia, in a cubicle in the emergency admissions unit, having soiled herself.

We got there about 10 o'clock and I could not believe my eyes. The door was wide open. There were people walking past. Mum was in bed with the cot sides up and she hadn't got a stitch of clothing on. I mean, she would have been horrified. She was completely naked and if I said covered in faeces, she was. It was everywhere. It was in her hair, her eyes, her nails, her hands and on all the cot sides, so she had obviously been trying to lift herself up or move about, because the bed was covered and it was literally everywhere and it was dried. It would have been there a long time. It wasn't new. (Francis, 2010, p. 57)

As separation from, and denial of, bodily failure and squalor become forever easier in the squeaky clean environments many of us in higher-income countries in the 21st century enjoy, it is easy to deny the inhumanity of nature. Most of us simply have little acquaintance with it. A generation of young adults have grown up who recoil from blood (post-HIV), change their clothes so often they do not know what body odour is, never come into contact with babies' nappies and have certainly never seen a dead body. As George Orwell wrote:

People talk about the horror of war, but what weapon has man invented that even approaches in cruelty some of the commoner diseases? 'Natural death' almost by definition means something slow, smelly and painful. (Orwell, 1946)

While many of the diseases Orwell was referring to have been eradicated in countries like the UK, there is no escaping the vicissitudes of the flesh. Raymond Tallis, British philosopher and retired professor of geriatric medicine, comments on the enormity in the history of civilisation of the imaginative and moral step involved in engaging with the realities of illness. He describes a challenging process of *cognitive self-overcoming* on the part of humanity and reminds us that humans found it easier to assume an objective attitude towards the stars than towards their own inner organs (Tallis, 2005, p. 13). This self-overcoming – surely one of humanity's greatest achievements – has to be done on an individual level by thousands of NHS staff every day as they muster the will, the necessary balance of kindness and professional detachment, to perform the most intimate tasks imaginable. No wonder they struggle sometimes to manage and process their feelings – and no wonder that they can fall short of attentive, kind and attuned care.

Contact with emotional distress and disturbance can be equally, if not more, harrowing. Existential questions about identity, suffering and death are raised and may put people in touch with extreme feelings of pain and loss. The struggle with feelings of helplessness and hopelessness in the face of suffering cannot be avoided, although different people cope in very different ways. A workshop participant quoted by Firth-Cozens & Cornwell (2009, p. 6) commented as follows:

I went to work on an elderly ward where patients died daily and there was great pressure on beds. At first I did all I could to make the lead up to death have some meaning and to feel something when one of them died. But gradually the number of deaths and the need to strip down beds and get another patient in as fast as you can got to me and I became numb to the patients; it became just about the rate of turnover, nothing else.

There has recently been a spate of articles in the British press about high sickness rates among NHS staff (10.7 days per employee each year in 2009) compared with the average worker in the private sector (6.4 days per employee each year) and the possible link with high levels of unhealthy habits such as smoking and with obesity. Surprisingly, the focus in many parts of the press was the alleged hypocrisy and double standards of healthcare staff, while any possible link with the distressing nature of the work was largely ignored.

Engaging with ill-being

Staying open to the needs and experience of the patient in the face of one's own motivations and reactions to illness is essentially a psychological task. Modern healthcare policy and guidance makes frequent reference to the notion of working to promote the patient's *well-being*. This concept involves more than symptom management, reduction or cure. It is about how a patient is *in him/herself* and *in his/her environment*, including relationships, roles and activities, and meaningful inclusion in the world. It is worth considering the opposite concept: that of *ill-being*. Ill-being is more than symptoms and disease, and it is what healthcare workers meet most of the time. It is important to understand what this encounter is like, how it impinges on healthcare work and how it might influence a sense of kinship and the expression of kindness.

Ill-being is a state of *complex unease* in oneself and in one's environment. A person may find it hard to name, evaluate or express the basic symptoms of an illness. Those symptoms will, themselves, interfere with relationships, roles and responsibilities, with emotional consequences – for the patient and those around them. The symptoms, or the very name of an illness, may evoke complex mixtures of guilt, shame, anger, victimhood or fear – in the patient and in others. Symptoms, or the illness itself, may provoke denial and flight – again in the sufferer or kin. There may be highly charged cultural or political dimensions to an illness, or to its care and treatment; examples include complex healthcare problems in the offspring of cousin marriages in various communities, HIV in the gay community and the stigma of mental illness. Public fears and agitation about such illnesses as 'epidemic' flu and BSE bring another dimension to the uneasy state of ill-being, and to the healthcare worker's relationship with it. Patients may be well aware of many of the dimensions of their ill-being, vaguely aware of others and completely unconscious of yet other responses to their situation.

Healthcare workers must manage to engage with and 'read through' these many dimensions of ill-being. They must join the patient in this uneasy and uncertain state to begin to empathise, to evaluate and to respond. The process of diagnosis, frequently complex and uncertain, is complicated and coloured by the nature of ill-being. Continued empathic attention and response are challenging in this state of joint unease. Often the patient's ill-being will evoke difficult feelings in the worker, sometimes in very obvious ways, like felt disapproval, overprotectiveness, anger or fear, and sometimes more obscurely, with subtler disturbances to engagement, empathy or response. Being intelligently kind in these circumstances requires self-awareness and the capacity to manage oneself in one's role.

Psychological defence mechanisms

One of the important themes in this book is the idea that we need to think more about how to help people process disturbing feelings generated by healthcare work. The concept of *psychological defence mechanisms* is helpful here. This is a model for understanding how an individual mind protects itself from being overwhelmed. The fundamental process is that of *repression*, where thoughts and feelings that threaten because of their disturbing nature are shut out of consciousness. This shutting out happens without our awareness, and is achieved through using defence mechanisms. Some of the more common defence mechanisms are briefly summarised below.

- *Displacement* involves the redirection of our feelings towards people or things that are not the cause of them, but which are easier to deal with – the 'kicking the cat' phenomenon.
- In *projection* we ascribe our feelings to others instead of struggling with them ourselves – through such processes as scapegoating or infantilising other people, we get the chance to deal with bad or dependent feelings by ascribing them to the other.
- *Rationalisation* leads to us inventing reasons for our feelings and behaviour more comfortable to us than the real ones – an example would be 'I did it for your own good' – and can be closely related to *minimisation* – 'it was only a little punch'.
- In *reaction formation*, anxiety-provoking or unacceptable emotions and impulses are mastered by exaggeration of the directly opposing tendency – hence our discomfort with showy, sentimental, ingratiating expressions of 'love', and the often used quote from *Hamlet* – 'the lady doth protest too much, methinks'.
- *Sublimation* is when the energy attached to an unacceptable or destructive impulse is converted into a creative or more acceptable activity – the sublimation of aggression into, for example, positive promotion of professional interests and perspectives, such as union activity, or, in personal life, into a sporting activity.

These and other defence mechanisms evoke intuitive recognition in most of us, even in people who do not subscribe to the full psychoanalytic view of the world. Some of these mechanisms are illustrated in what follows. The point, though, is that they are happening, to some extent or the other, all the time: life is a complex drama, with complicated subplots involving combinations of these ways of defending ourselves from its complexity and pain. Sometimes we can recognise that these things are happening – in ourselves or others – but at other times we are quite unaware.

We all use defence mechanisms, so they do not in themselves indicate pathology. Indeed, like the inflammatory response, they can be understood as a defence system that in many situations protects and promotes survival. But just as smoking and overeating are examples of coping mechanisms that have become problems in themselves, so mental defence mechanisms, if overused or extreme, will become rigid shells which narrow our personality and capacity to relate to others. In extreme cases, the behaviours driven by the defence mechanism take over as the focus of the problem and become part of a vicious circle from which it is hard to escape.

Because healthcare work is so emotionally demanding, defence mechanisms will be evoked frequently. Individuals, depending on their personality and past experience, will protect themselves in different ways from the emotionally traumatic environment. A group of doctors and nurses working in an emergency department, for example, involved in managing the casualties of a severe road traffic accident, might manage the feelings engendered in very different ways. One might cope with her feeling of helplessness by being unnecessarily bossy; another will go straight off to the library and bury himself in intellectual work; another will go partying and tell over-the-top jokes all night; yet another will take her anger out on her husband, arguing over something trivial. While these are all legitimate and understandably human ways of coping in the short term with a virtually unbearable experience, problems can arise if staff are exposed to frequent emotional trauma, without space to process their feelings. Defensive styles of coping then become entrenched. As walls build up, feelings of vulnerability and sadness become more deeply buried. Kindness suffers as the capacity for fellow feeling recedes.

Over-identification

Even emotionally well-supported staff used to managing traumatising situations may find that a particular incident or patient gets under their skin and throws them into turmoil. This may be because the situation resonates with their own experiences in a way that might not even be conscious at the time. Peter Speck, a hospital chaplain, used to working with death and the dying, described the tragic death of a 13-year-old boy who had run in front of a lorry because he was late for school (Speck, 1994). Speck describes candidly how the level of his own distress prevented him being of much support to the parents and his over-identification was such that he even mixed up the name of the dying boy, John, with his own son, David. Once Speck had been helped to reflect on the level of his upset and work out what was going on in his mind, he was able to resume his role and be emotionally available to the suffering parents.

Then I remembered how that morning, as I was leaving for work, I had heard my wife shouting up to our son 'you're late! Get out of bed, now!' When Mrs Brown had used exactly these words in telling me her story, she momentarily became my own wife, telling me that our son was dying. (Speck, 1994, p. 95)

Kindness is rooted in fellow feeling, a sense of the other as kith and kin, yet here is an example of over-identification being unhelpful. In healthcare, there will always be patients who resemble ourselves or people who are especially significant to us. This brings the work 'closer to home' and can cut through the defences we have built up. Sometimes it can feel a relief to be more connected; at others, the experience can feel unbearable. In the story described by Speck, the important point is that he was able to become consciously aware of how his mind was working and understand why he was behaving in the way he did. This psychological work enabled him to untangle the muddle between his own family situation and the Brown family, which was interfering with his capacity to help them. It is easy to imagine how some staff might have reacted to an experience like this by distancing themselves in an attempt to prevent similar situations in the future from touching them in the same way.

Linked to the concept of empathy is the idea that there is an optimal emotional distance from the work that can both help sustain one's own well-being and allow one to be emotionally helpful to patients. Of course, this is an ideal, best envisaged as a rough line which needs to be kept in mind as one swings above and below it and struggles to return to it. Problems arise if one becomes fixed too far from this line and unable to get back.

Guilt and self-blame

Over-identification is just one of many situations that can trigger extreme anxiety in healthcare work. Another is the feeling of guilt and the capacity for self-blame. These feelings may be aroused irrationally by distressing, but unavoidable, 'failures' of treatment – despite one's best efforts, someone suffers or dies. More rarely, real mistakes are made. This is inevitable in a field of such complexity and inherent pressures but nevertheless can haunt the individuals involved for years. Being part of intricate interventions where the outcome is frequently life or death can be experienced as an unbearably heavy burden, whether there are mistakes or not.

Medical life is dogged by a sense of inadequacy, by guilt and self-blame. When a patient dies and one believes, rightly or wrongly, that he might have been saved had things been managed differently, one is put into the role of a guilty survivor. The usual reassurances ... seem obscenely inadequate to such a despair. A death cannot be glossed over by Christmas-cracker aphorisms. Doctors who make mistakes feel frightened, guilty and alone. (Tallis, 2005, p. 213)

Many would say the loneliness Tallis refers to has got worse over the past two decades, as the likelihood – or fear – of litigation makes it difficult to share one's doubts with colleagues. Efforts have been made to reverse the culture of individual blame and focus instead on systemic failures. In practice, though, many healthcare staff suffer terribly at the thought that they might have contributed in some way to a death and live in dread of making a mistake and being publicly humiliated. The media, with its readiness to churn out scare stories about the NHS and its staff in an increasingly contemptuous tone, does nothing to help matters. And more generally, our attitude to risk as a society and the perception that anything that goes wrong – including death – must be someone's fault affect everyone.

One of the things that keeps clinical staff awake at night is the amount of uncertainty involved in the job. Inevitably, given the complexity of the human body, the art of medicine and healthcare is about managing uncertainty with the best interest of the patient in mind; uncertainty is the rule rather than the exception. This means that, on a day-by-day basis, clinicians are sifting evidence and experience, signs and symptoms in the patient and making irreversible, often life or death, decisions based on best probabilities. Add to this the inevitable reality that such decisions often have to be made quickly, under huge pressure, and it is not difficult to understand why staff are often worn down and preoccupied by nagging doubts and a sense of failure. And remember, too, that many are unconsciously driven to do the job by a need for reparation because of early experiences only partly understood – what has been termed *the self-assigned impossible task* (Zagier Roberts, 1994, p. 110). This makes it particularly difficult to distinguish between failing someone in a particular circumstance and *being* a failure.

On a less dramatic level, the culture of competition and performance management, while providing more opportunities for individuals to reach their potential, also raises the fear of failure. Some would argue that the inherent drivers in healthcare are sufficient and too much performance management – particularly if it is clumsily implemented – risks pushing already highly driven and stressed-out staff to anxiety levels way above the optimum. This raised anxiety may paradoxically cause them to be more defensive and less emotionally available – with the obvious consequences for patient satisfaction and clinical outcomes.

The need to manage feelings of anger and hatred

One aspect of guilt which staff tend to find uncomfortable and difficult to talk about is the guilt generated by feelings of anger towards, or strong dislike or even hatred of a patient. Patients can be rude and very demanding, particularly when they are frightened, confused and in pain. Staff surveys have shown how common it is for staff to be physically abused, threatened and denigrated. Nowadays, there are signs in most wards and out-patient units warning of a 'zero tolerance' stance to any threatening behaviour towards staff. Such policies are simplistic and over-generalised. They may protect staff from some of the grosser forms of behaviour but they allow little room for the effects of disease, disorientation and fear, and therefore the policies they announce need a wide margin of discretion when they are implemented. Occasionally, staff are left physically hurt by patients (or, very rarely indeed, the victim of a homicide), but a much higher proportion are left emotionally traumatised and mistrustful. Many feel that their altruism has been betrayed and make efforts, consciously or unconsciously, to protect themselves better in the future.

There are many reasons to dislike a patient, some more understandable than others. It is all too easy to feel furious with patients who appear to be undermining all efforts to help them. Some patient groups are seen as undeserving, such as people who have harmed themselves or fallen over in a drunken stupor (Hughes & Kosky, 2007). Understandably, staff on a medical ward or in a frantically busy emergency department may find it difficult to nurse a teenager who has overdosed if they also have to care for an acutely ill patient with heart failure. However, staff report feeling much more compassionate towards people who harm themselves if they have had some input to help them reflect on why people behave in this manner and a safe forum to express their feelings, including frustration and anger – and sometimes sheer dislike. Even within psychiatry, there is often a kind of unacknowledged hierarchy, with these patient groups seen as less deserving than others with a more clear-cut illness, such as schizophrenia.

Individual staff are particularly prone to suffer from guilt and depression if their hateful feelings towards a patient are not shared by the rest of the team or feel so unacceptable that they are kept from conscious awareness. It may be that the individual is in touch with a hateful part of the patient that others in the team are not being exposed to. Or it may be that the patient's situation or personality reminds the staff member of something they find hard to manage in their own life – their mother's tendency to helplessness perhaps, or their father's cold manner. These types of resonances are inevitable but often feel unacceptable, particularly to nursing staff driven by the idea of themselves as angelic carers. Hateful feelings driven by fear of disease and suffering, the physical disgust described above, and a sense of being way out of one's depth can also be difficult to face.

The need to manage dependency and loneliness

While scandals involving a few clinicians and their improper relations with patients are the cause of many of the inquiries conducted by the General Medical Council (GMC), these sexual liaisons point to a wider issue, relating to the need for comfort and closeness, and the management of boundaries. Healthcare has at its heart, however much we speak of 'empowering the patient', the issue of dependency. The patient depends on the clinician's goodwill, kindness and skill, and the clinician may well be unconsciously depending on the patient (through getting well) to make them feel good and well in return. The experience of the patient can feel very lonely – and often clinicians will be experiencing their own form of loneliness. In this 'mutual loneliness' either or both in this relationship may begin to see in the other someone to meet needs that are personal and beyond the terms of the working relationship. The most dramatic form of this response may be sexual, but there are other ways in which too close, and too dependent, a relationship can express itself. Each may idealise the other, and the wish not to disappoint the other may skew communication, honesty and the interactions of caregiver and patient. The disappointment inherent in managing these feelings may, of course, tip over into anger and hostility.

Dependency and vulnerability are frightening states of mind. One response can be to denigrate such feelings, to regard them as demeaning, 'pathetic' or worse. Many healthcare workers are loath to acknowledge these emotions or situations in themselves. They may deny them, and begin to work in isolated anxiety and exhaustion. Another reaction is to 'collapse' into self-pity when the feelings finally break through. Rather more sinister, though, can be the phenomenon of holding sick patients in contempt for their neediness, even to hate them for it. Many patently kind people will admit to the occasional intrusion of such feelings – especially those who care for people with long-term debilitating conditions. Others will not feel it safe to voice such feelings, a situation that is likely to harm themselves and their patients.

Being good enough rather than perfect

The majority of healthcare staff suffer from anxiety on and off throughout their career, sometimes at a level which makes life difficult (Firth-Cozens, 2003). Depersonalisation is often a component of severe stress and burnout and will limit kindness or even, at the extreme, produce cruelty. Clinical depression is common among healthcare workers and higher than in the general population (Caplan, 1994; Wall *et al*, 1997). Feelings of guilt and humiliation, helplessness in the face of suffering and fear of making mistakes predominate, as do negative mental states to do with self-blame and inadequacy. While some staff end up having to take significant periods of sick leave or retire, others keep working, often for years. Self-absorption (often linked with self-protection) is another feature of depression – and the result of this combination of feelings is that the capacity for kindness is inevitably affected.

The idea of being *good enough* can be a lifeline. This is an expression first coined by Donald Winnicott (1965), who was both a paediatrician and a psychoanalyst and delivered a series of popular radio talks to mothers in the kindly, rather paternalistic fashion of the day. Winnicott reassured mothers not only that they did not need to be perfect and that being merely *good enough* was all right, but that in fact their babies' mental development depended on them *not* trying to fulfil their babies' every need. In other words, experiencing minimal frustration – ideally in manageable rather than traumatising chunks – is important for the process of individuation.

This idea is particularly helpful in the field of mental health, where new staff have a tendency in some areas to think that unconditional love will cure all, unwittingly infantilising the patients in the process. More generally, being 'good enough' is the only realistic aspiration for staff who want to avoid burnout. Being 'good enough' is not about shrugging one's shoulders in an offhand manner when standards are not met. It is more about letting go of the idea that everything is down to oneself as an individual. Being good enough depends on good teamwork. It also links to the important idea that adopting a kind and compassionate attitude to oneself is a prerequisite for being kind to others.

Compassionate mind training

An exciting new development over recent years has been a scientific interest in *mindfulness* and the growing understanding of the role of positive emotions in sustaining mental health and well-being. A specific application of this is 'compassionate mind training' (CMT), an intervention that is attracting increasing interest within the field of mental health (Gilbert, 2009). The principles behind this are drawn from a wide range of fields, including evolutionary psychology, neuroscience and models of emotion, cognition and behaviour – some of which will be explored in later chapters of this book.

CMT refers to the specific techniques that can be used to help us experience compassion and to develop various aspects of compassion towards ourselves and others. Compassion includes attributes and skills and is best understood as a pattern of organising these various components of the mind. If you are feeling under threat, for example, it is likely that the compassionate components of your mind are turned off and instead your mind has a pattern of motivation and ways of feeling that are about protecting yourself from danger. In CMT, one practises activating the components of compassion such that they organise and pattern the mind in certain ways. The idea is to change one's relationship to emerging thoughts and feelings rather than to change the thoughts themselves. Empathy for one's own distress, for example, is fundamental.

Of course, the aspiration to develop a more compassionate state of mind is not new: the techniques are adapted from Buddhism and link to the practice of meditative prayer in other religions. It is not straightforward and for some people will involve working with a lot of anxious ambivalence towards compassion – particularly self-compassion, which can feel frighteningly unfamiliar in our frenetic, acquisitive, 21st-century environment.

Michael Sandel, Harvard Professor of Government, argues that virtues such as altruism and fellow feeling are 'like muscles that develop and grow stronger with exercise' (Sandel, 2009). If we accept that prioritising kindness and kinship is important, we need to find ways of facilitating this 'exercise'. CMT is accessible and relatively easily taught. It would not be impractical to include this type of training in professional curricula or to give everyone the opportunity to do this training as part of continuing professional development. Pilot studies could be evaluated from various perspectives, looking, for example, at the effects on the individual staff member, patient experience, team morale and organisational efficiency. There is clearly the potential for making a positive impact on the virtuous circle described in Chapter 3.

The culture of training and education

More generally, individual workers and professions need to reinstate attentive kindness as a central and valued professional quality and skill – and to restore kindness to its pre-eminent place in the 'duty of care'. This will involve radical attention to recruitment, education and training. At the heart of all professional development must be placed the capacity to make and sustain attentive relationships with patients, because this is as important as any theoretical or technical education. The ability to pay attention, to empathise with and make sense of patient need and experience requires self-management and commitment, and needs to be practised in an ongoing way if it is to be sustained under pressure. *Attentive relating* to patients needs to be recognised as a complex but fundamental psychosocial skill. Like all complex social skills, it involves understanding both oneself and others, and needs to be learned through experience. Only if staff are helped to recognise the effects on themselves of patient ill-being and the healthcare task itself will such capability develop.

The culture of education and training would benefit from consideration of these aims. A mixture of financial pressures, and the sheer problems of releasing staff, make training and development a challenge for NHS organisations. The twin drivers of regulation and risk aversion (associated with feared financial penalties) have led to a proliferation of 'statutory' and 'mandatory' training. The training, though, is frequently indiscriminate. It is common for a business planner and a nurse both to do the same 'handling and lifting' course – every year; an expert on child protection and domestic violence sits alongside her secretary for the same annual whistle-stop tour of child protection. Frequently there are duplications between statutory and mandatory training. No one questions whether annually is right – it just is. And if you come in from another trust you must do most of it again so that regulation can be satisfied. There is an enormous opportunity to rethink this kind of training – to ensure the right people get the right training at the right level, to remove duplication, to consider frequency and so on. The opportunity to free up money and time to enable the creation of a learning environment to nourish kindness in practice is obvious.

Though the current vogue for 'competencies' has some value, an approach that educates and nurtures intelligent kindness cannot simply concern whether people know about and can do things. 'Applied' compassionate care depends on internalising values, empathy, the capacity to communicate kindness and concern, and the ability to maintain an attentive frame of mind in difficult circumstances. These things are *human qualities* rather than competencies. There has been a trend, in nursing education particularly, for training to become more academic, with a focus on the technical aspects of physical care and less attention to conduct and interpersonal aspects of care (Chambers & Ryder, 2009, p. 13). To support the development of intelligent kindness, clinical educators need to build a culture of reflection and enquiry and provide a living–learning experience that promotes self-awareness and learning from mistakes.

An effective medium for nurturing intelligent kindness would ensure that students, trainees and experienced workers alike receive sensitive and on-going feedback – some of it directly from patients. This would form part of an ongoing reflective dialogue as to how they are operating as people in their roles, a dialogue that should continue throughout a career. While healthcare courses tend to include psychosocial and ethics components, too often such initiatives are one-off courses or discussions, token gestures, rather than being integral to the whole of healthcare. As such, they are too easily seen by trainees as irrelevant (Wear & Zarconi, 2008).

In the King's Fund 'Point of Care' report on enabling compassionate care, Firth-Cozens & Cornwell (2009, p. 10) identify two important components of teaching compassion. The first is *getting close to the patient*. It is the present authors' experience that trainee psychiatric professionals, when they encounter real patient stories, especially if the patient is actually speaking, find it a particularly memorable educational experience. As Firth-Cozens & Cornwell point out, many health professionals have also been patients or have had someone close become a patient and such experiences can be usefully shared. Some medical schools include family placements in the undergraduate curriculum, where students are allocated to, and make regular visits to, a family struggling with some form of chronic disability or disorder.

The second component Firth-Cozens & Cornwall pick out as important in the development of healthcare professionals is *role modelling*. It is clear that role models, good and bad, have an impact. Early impressions stay with us, and there is a tendency to internalise values and to emulate the mannerisms of those we admire, often without even being aware we are doing so. The unconscious nature of imitation has been supported by the discovery of *mirror neurons*; these have been shown to fire not only when we perform an action, but also when we observe an action performed by someone else –

so-called 'motor empathy' (Rizzolatti & Craighero, 2004). Unfortunately, there is some evidence that 'bad' role models tend to be as powerful as 'good' ones (Sinclair, 1997). This may be because the defence mechanisms they deploy – often of a grandiose, omnipotent, manic nature – appear an attractive short-cut to trainees struggling with painful anxiety and conflict.

Most importantly, trainees need to feel kindly treated themselves and part of a culture where kindness is valued and modelled. All trainees should have a personal tutor or mentor, where an explicit part of the role is to be attentive to the trainee's experience, and to model and encourage an attitude of intelligent kindness. More generally, there needs to be greater understanding that kindness to patients will be more sustainable if staff are self-aware and able to treat themselves kindly. This needs to extend through practical issues such as ensuring staff get proper breaks to noticing signs of stress and upset and making enough space to give the extra support needed when things are particularly difficult. Although the experience of compassion can feel painful, tackling problems and talking about them are associated with lower stress levels (Koeske et al, 1993) and, provided the appropriate support is in place, can improve psychological well-being (Post, 2005).

Supervision and support

Undoubtedly, many healthcare staff have to struggle with situations that take them to the brink of their humanity and modern pressures may exacerbate this. The culture of the modern health service is frequently poorly suited to the emotional labour involved in effectively containing such anxiety. The importance of such work is poorly recognised, and the skills and attention of leaders are not directed to addressing this need.

Despite lip service being paid to the importance of supervision, this is not yet sufficiently valued and prioritised in the NHS. It is unusual for individuals to feel that they have been helped to consider their general experience of the work, let alone identify and cope with deep-seated fears, in a way that develops their capacity for consciously managing the psychological demands associated with the task. The current bias towards monitoring performance, implementing procedures and developing competencies through supervision requires a clear shift. It would be productive if supervision were to concentrate much more on helping staff to manage themselves in their roles, process difficult feelings, sustain compassionate attention and develop the responsiveness and confidence to work with others to address patient need.

In everybody's training and ongoing practice there should be assistance in learning to recognise and work with such processes, including leaders and managers at the top of the organisation and support staff such as receptionists and porters. This is not a naïve argument for expensive and time-consuming reflective space, as the apparent expense and amount of time would be minimal compared with the effects of continuing to neglect these issues. Group supervision can also be useful – not just as an economic recourse, but as a way of creating a wider team and social milieu which nourishes kindness in practice.

The interplay between the individual, the team and the organisation is vital to the theme of this book. For if, as a society, we want a workforce who feel secure enough to invest deeply in the work, to put patients before self-interest, to be sufficiently in touch with their own vulnerability to show compassion towards the suffering of others, then we need to think about the type of culture we wish to create. We need constantly to look for ways to make it more secure, consistent and affirming. One dimension of this is the direct and clear affirmation that kindness and compassion should be actively nurtured, as captured in this quote from the King's Fund:

Like high stress levels, a lack of compassion too flows through teams and organizations rather than just occurring in occasional dyads; the opposite is also true – providing kindnesses to staff will enable more to reach patients. (Firth-Cozens & Cornwell, 2009, p. 11)

Contrast this with the reports from staff in the Mid-Staffordshire inquiry of the prevalent bullying, the rudeness and hostility, the lack of support and general climate of fear – for example, the words of a medical consultant about how he saw the nurses being treated:

I got no sense that the nurses had any protection whatsoever. I felt that nurses were hung out within the department. They were definitely not supported. (Francis, 2010, p. 188)

It is really very simple: the safer people feel in their role, the more they will be able to look with curiosity at their own attitudes and prejudices and be more open to the emotional experience of their patients.

References

Caplan, R. P. (1994) Stress, anxiety and depression in hospital consultants, general practitioners and senior health managers. *BMJ*, **335**, 184–187.

Chambers, C. & Ryder, E. (2009) *Compassion and Care in Nursing*. Radcliffe.

Farquharson, G. (2004) How good staff become bad. In *From Toxic Institutions to Therapeutic Environments* (eds P. Campling, S. Davies & G. Farquharson), pp. 12–19. Gaskell.

Firth-Cozens, J. (2003) Doctors, their wellbeing, and their stress. *BMJ*, **326**, 670–671.

Firth-Cozens, J. & Cornwell, J. (2009) *The Point of Care. Enabling Compassionate Care in Acute Hospital Settings*. King's Fund.

Francis, R. (2010) *The Independent Inquiry into Care Provided by Mid-Staffordshire NHS Foundation Trust, January 2005–March 2009*. HMSO.

Gilbert, P. (2009) *The Compassionate Mind: A New Approach to Life's Challenges*. Constable and Robinson.

Hughes, L. & Kosky, N. (2007) Meeting NICE self-harm standards in an accident and emergency department. *The Psychiatrist*, **31**, 255–258.

Jones, A. M. (2010) Could kindness heal the NHS? *BMJ*, **340**, c3166.

Koeske, G. F., Kirk, S. A. & Koeske, R. D. (1993) Coping with job stress: which strategies work best? *Journal of Occupational and Organizational Psychology*, **66**, 319–335.

Lowenstein, J. (2008) *The Midnight Meal and Other Essays About Doctors, Patients and Medicine.* Yale University Press.

Orwell, G. (1946) How the poor die. In *The Collected Essays, Journalism and Letters of George Orwell. Vol. 4: In Front of Your Nose, 1945–50* (eds S. Orwell & I. Angus), pp. 261–272. Penguin (1970).

Patients Association (2010) *Patients Not Numbers. People Not Statistics.* Patients Association.

Post, S. G. (2005) Altruism, happiness and health: it's good to be good. *International Journal of Behavioural Medicine*, **12**, 66–77.

Rizzolatti, G. & Craighero, L. (2004) The mirror-neuron system. *Annual Review of Neuroscience*, **27**, 169–172.

Sandel, M. (2009) Reith Lectures 2009, Lecture 4: 'Politics of the common good', broadcast 30 June, Radio 4.

Sinclair, S. (1997) *Making Doctors.* Berg.

Speck, P. (1994) Working with dying people. In *The Unconscious at Work* (eds A.Obholzer & V. Zagier Roberts), pp. 94–100. Brunner–Routledge.

Tallis, R. (2005) *Hippocratic Oaths: Medicine and Its Discontents.* Atlantic Books.

Wall, T. D., Bolden, R. I., Borrill, C. S., *et al* (1997) Minor psychiatric disorder in NHS staff: occupational and gender differences. *British Journal of Psychiatry*, **171**, 519–523.

Wear, D. & Zarconi, J. (2008) Can compassion be taught? Let's ask the students. *Journal of General Internal Medicine*, **23**, 948–953.

Winnicott, D. W. (1965) *The Maturational Processes and the Facilitating Environment.* International Universities Press.

Zagier Roberts, V. (1994) The self-assigned impossible task. In *The Unconscious at Work* (eds A.Obholzer & V. Zagier Roberts), pp. 110–118. Brunner–Routledge.

CHAPTER 5

The emotional life of teams

Insanity in individuals is something rare; in nations, groups, parties and epochs it is the rule. (Nietzsche)

The team dynamic

Ideally, the work people do should bring out the best in them. This does not always happen. The previous chapter explored some of the reasons why individuals can find it hard to provide compassionate healthcare. This chapter is about group dynamics: how people behave in teams, but also how teams behave in relation to other teams.

Most of us have some awareness that our behaviour can be affected by the group of people we are with, that working in a 'good' team is a very different experience from working in a 'bad' team. We may even have caught ourselves behaving 'out of character' in a particular group situation, or celebrated having the 'best brought out of us' in another. Being part of a group or team can provoke anxiety. We want to feel accepted and liked but also to retain our sense of individuality. We prefer to see ourselves as autonomous and the agents of control in our lives but have some awareness that our thoughts and feelings are heavily influenced, often to a surprising degree. We are most conscious of this anxiety when we are new to a particular team. Then we may catch ourselves sizing up the other members, wondering how we shall fit in, looking for similarities and differences, trying to work out the official hierarchies and professional divisions as well as where the real power lies and the informal subgroupings that might form around things such as age, race or hobbies.

Healthcare teams tend to draw from a wide spectrum of society in terms of race, religion, age, socioeconomic status, educational achievement and personality types – with all the richness that such diversity brings. But such diversity can also lead to tensions around difference, which can be amplified when everyone is under pressure. Underneath all this, we may be vaguely conscious of more intuitive stirrings of trust and mistrust, sexual attraction and repulsion, fear, competitiveness and shadowy resonances with other people and situations, particularly teams we have worked with in the past. As these develop into rivalries, romances, subgroupings and so on, the potential for being emotionally available for the task in hand will be affected.

In the main, there is a tendency to underestimate the effect of the group and a poor understanding of how group dynamics can influence behaviour. This is an area where centuries of accumulated wisdom and decades of research and theoretical understanding have made little impact on the general consciousness. In the Western world, where personal autonomy is valued so highly, it is uncomfortable to think of behaviour being driven by – often unconscious – group forces.

If we are serious about the importance of kindness, there is a need to understand how it can be facilitated or undermined by the group dynamic. In the aftermath of the Second World War, people were asking a much more extreme version of this question as they tried to come to terms with the atrocities committed – the industrial scale of sadistic death systems in place and the widespread collusion. The human capacity for treating others cruelly has much preoccupied thinkers in the years since, but hardly gets a mention in health professional curricula. A number of instructive, classic experiments from social science and psychology have famously demonstrated how easy it is to impair an individual's capacity for independent thought and moral judgement and illustrate the universality of the problem.

Group pressure

The first experiment, by Solomon Asch (1951), showed the powerful capacity of the group to undermine individuals' belief in the information that they are receiving from their senses and the overwhelming inclination in most of us to conform to the group. His study involved groups of nine people, only one of whom was a real volunteer participant: the rest were confederates of the experimenter. Groups were asked to make judgements in a series of questions comparing different lines in a diagram. Once the experiment got going, the eight confederates would give wrong answers and the effect that this had on the responses of the genuine participants was monitored. Overall, 76% made at least one error, compared with 99% accuracy in pre-tests where no one had been planted to give deliberately wrong answers.

Many of the participants argued afterwards that they conformed only because they did not want to stand out from the group (i.e. they claimed to know they were giving the wrong answer) but even when this possibility was eliminated by changing the experiment so that other group members were unable to see the answers of the participant and judge them, the error rate was significant. This suggests that *beliefs themselves* were influenced by simply being in the presence of others with seemingly different beliefs as well as there being strong pressures to conform. Very few of the participants in this study were able to stand up against the prevailing group opinion, despite the evidence of their own eyes. This experiment has been repeated in numerous studies since, with similar results (Bond & Smith, 1996).

Such research has direct relevance to our understanding of institutions and the sometimes inhumane behaviour of those who work in them. Although 'closed' institutions, such as secure units, are particularly vulnerable, all health services workers are susceptible to the process of institutionalisation, where the capacity to think independently becomes weakened by group pressure. This is one of the themes of the report of the Mid-Staffordshire inquiry: 'there was an acceptance of standards of care, probably through habituation, that should not have been tolerated' (Francis, 2010, p. 86). An interesting phenomenon in the Mid-Staffordshire inquiry was how 'disappointingly few' staff were willing to give independent evidence (p. 31). This would be partly down to a sense of loyalty or fear, but there is a suggestion that individuals were also confused about what they thought.

I also held a series of meetings for staff at the hospital.... Some of these were attended by a very small number. It was clear to me that some of those, in particular nursing staff, were very hesitant to express views which they feared might be considered disloyal to their employer, if those views came to the Trust's attention. A phrase commonly used was 'I cannot believe I am saying this.' (p. 34)

Our relationship to authority

In another major series of (now rather distasteful) experiments, by Stanley Milgram (1963), the participants – ordinary people – were told that the experimenters were exploring the effects of punishment on learning. They were instructed to apply increasingly powerful electric shocks, rising to 450 volts, to apparent 'students' in response to a failure to learn a task. Despite seeing the physical distress caused by the electric shocks (in fact feigned by the 'students' but seen as real by the participants), most of the participants continued to do as they were told, when, despite their questions, and in some cases upset and protest, they were sternly instructed to continue. The physical distress observed escalated from the apparent victims of this regime banging on the walls, to complaining about their heart condition and eventually to collapsing completely. The experiment is frequently cited as an example of how easily we succumb to the power of malignant authority.

Variations on the experiment have been carried out in many different countries and cultures, with the percentage of participants who are prepared to inflict fatal voltages remaining remarkably constant, at 61–66%, according to a meta-analysis (Blass, 2000). In general, where the victim's physical immediacy was increased, the participants' compliance decreased. The participants' compliance also decreased when the authority's physical immediacy decreased, for example if contact was over the telephone. The highest compliance was in experiments where the task of implementing the shocks was divided up and the participants presumably felt they were only small cogs in the system. In 2009, a version of the experiment was repeated as part of a television documentary entitled 'How violent are you?' (*Horizon*, BBC2). Of the 12 participants, only three refused to continue to the end of the experiment.

Conforming to role expectations

An experiment by Philip Zimbardo in the 1970s developed these themes. He devised an extended prison role situation where 24 students were randomly allocated to play the role of prisoner or guard. Despite being given no further instruction, the students took up extremely stereotypical roles and ended up with the guards adopting frankly sadistic behaviours while the prisoners became increasingly passive and depressed. So extreme was the distress experienced by some of the 'prisoners' that the experiment had to be stopped after 6 days rather than running for the planned 2 weeks. Moreover, some of the 'guards' were so gratified by the roles they were playing that they wanted to carry on for longer (Haney *et al*, 1973).

While the Milgram and Zimbardo series of experiments are of their time and would now be criticised on a number of accounts, not least ethical considerations, they speak for themselves in illustrating how easily ordinary people can be pulled into situations where they collude with or actively instigate not just unkind but frankly cruel, abusive behaviour. Interestingly, a version of Zimbardo's experiment was repeated more recently on the BBC in a documentary programme called *The Experiment* (see Reicher & Haslam, 2006). Perhaps in line with the way attitudes to authority and power have shifted over the past 30 years, the 'guards' were more lenient, but a group of 'prisoners' staged a coup and set up a regime where some of the others were badly treated and humiliated. Reicher & Haslam criticise many of the generalisations in the conclusion from the original Zimbardo experiment and specifically draw attention to the importance of leadership in the generation of institutional abuse.

These social psychology experiments illustrate: first, a tendency for the individual to conform to the group – to the degree that the group 'norm' is likely to override information from the individual's own sensory system; second, a tendency to obey authority figures – however dangerous; and third, a tendency to act into the roles expected of one – even if these involve cruelty. Interestingly, Zimbardo himself served as an expert witness for an Abu Ghraib defendant. The Abu Ghraib prison made international headlines in 2004 when photographs of military personnel abusing Iraqi prisoners were published. Much of the court proceedings focused on the general conditions in the prison, which were understood as contributing to the behaviour of the individuals on trial. While being clear that people are always accountable for their behaviour, Zimbardo believes that certain situations – and in this respect he said Abu Ghraib represented 'a perfect storm of conditions' (quoted on the website http://www.ted.com) – can be sufficiently powerful to undercut empathy, altruism and morality and make ordinary people commit horrendous acts. These insights cannot be dismissed. The capacity for groups of staff – be they in prisons, children's homes or hospitals – to participate in cruel and abusive regimes is ever evident. It is well to remember that such teams often have to face and process distress and disturbance that cannot be managed elsewhere in personal or community life.

Our hunter-gatherer heritage

An understanding of evolutionary history gives us another perspective on destructive group behaviours. Evolved design is not necessarily good design and an understanding of how human minds have evolved, and what they have evolved for, can offer valuable insights into the challenges of living and working together. Our brains are the result of millions of years of evolution and one way of understanding the psychological problems integral to modern life is to reflect on the brain's strategies as these reflect the range of emotions and social behaviours that are shared with our distant ancestors and many other animals. As one writer puts it, 'the passions and fears of the "old brain/mind" were designed to be very powerful and not easily over-ruled' (Gilbert, 2009, p. 36).

The hunter-gatherer lifestyle that existed for thousands of years made very different demands on the brain to life today. Hence our brains are designed to be threat-focused with a fast-acting system for alerting and protecting us from danger. This involves the hormone cortisol, which causes a generalised rise of anxiety and a rush of energy that can activate us to escape or fight or sometimes to freeze (the fright–fight–flight response).

In modern life, the sense of threat is prevalent but tends to be of a different kind and the response that evolution designed for our ancestors is often inappropriate and has to be inhibited. The fear and aggression experienced feel unwelcome and either are perceived as dysfunctional or are repressed and kept out of our conscious awareness. This leads to an overload of physiological symptoms, which in some cases leads to problems such as panic attacks, obsessive–compulsive symptoms and depression. While a neurophysiological system for soothing and comforting ourselves and each other has also evolved, the threat response – predominantly anger and fear – was designed to override these positive emotions in order to ensure survival. This is part of our evolutionary legacy.

Much social behaviour can be seen as driven by adaptive strategies to a primitive lifestyle that are not so adaptive to life in the 21st century. The tendency to compete for food and sex and to define ourselves as part of small groups – ideal for hunter-gatherers – can be seen as driving our relationships to a far greater extent than we are usually happy to acknowledge. This need to belong to small groups and feel connected can lead people to conform to group norms, split the world into insiders and outsiders, and institute social ranks and hierarchies, all of which can result in tribalism and hatred quite unhelpful to people leading modern lives as global citizens.

At a primitive level, it is in groups that human beings have to manage and express these passions and fears, and it is this that forms the basic material of group dynamics. Looking at the situation in the Mid-Stafford Trust through this lens, one can see the regressive tribalism that had resulted in the disengagement of managers and consultants, the hostile bullying culture that had perhaps arisen in the face of external threats (a huge financial deficit and punishing target culture) and how a compassionate mindset had been overridden in front-line staff by the threatening and poorly resourced culture they worked within.

The unconscious life of groups

Psychoanalytic thinking suggests that many of the things that happen in groups, many of the aspects of how well they work, are influenced by unconscious processes. People bring conflicting needs and desires into groups. How these things are played out and managed influences much of how a group feels and behaves. Groups – teams – struggle with several sources of conflict. Individuals want both autonomy and to be dependent on others. There is a tension between attending to the needs of the group for the group's sake, and to meeting the needs of its individual members. The team can be torn between investing collective effort or sitting back and expecting intense, often polarised work between a powerful pair of individuals within the group, to relieve everyone of responsibility for working with the complexity of the real world.

Wilfrid Bion suggests that how these conflicts are managed at any time leads the group to fall into one of three modes in which group feeling and behaviour appear to be based on an unconscious *basic assumption*:

- When the unconscious assumption is that the group's primary task is to meet people's *dependency* needs, its behaviour is typified by passivity, self-gratification and reliance on authority.
- When the assumption is that *fight–(or)–flight* is required to preserve autonomy, meet needs and escape difficulties, the group is characterised by conflict, especially with authority, by self-protection, by 'fleeing' from challenges in the task.
- When the assumption is that the *pairing* of powerful individuals will resolve group problems and needs, the group tends to sit back and invest their hope in magical solutions emerging in the future, rather than whole-group, 'adult' application to the challenges of the task in the present.

Bion thought that groups and teams can function in a fully engaged and creative 'work group' mode, but believed that they were in and out of one or other of these basic assumption states for short or long periods of time (Bion, 1961).

Reflection on experiences of being in teams may well prompt recognition of some of the ways Bion describes group psychology and behaviour – such patterns are also often vividly present in the relationship between a team and its wider environment. As important here as the specifics of the theory is Bion's highlighting of the contrast between a well-functioning, task-focused group and group behaviour that can, without conscious intention, fall into less than creative states. Ideas like Bion's prompt team members, and their leaders, to be attentive to the climate and culture of teams, 'how they are going about things', and to think about how best to move into effective 'work group' mode. They prompt team members to think about how they and their colleagues are collectively managing anxiety, their own needs, authority and the challenges of the task. When teams are in modes where self-gratification, passivity, conflict and evasion, or unrealistic expectation undermine attention to their task, they become vulnerable to poor functioning. Depending on the personalities of their members, and the anxieties and pressures of the task, this under-functioning can veer from understandable temporary distraction to more extreme states, where colleagues and patients are not met as persons.

Primitive defence mechanisms

We are all subject to group dynamics, even at the best of times, but some team settings evoke more extreme processes. The combination of an inherently traumatic and conflictual primary task, the close and complex working relationships that characterise a healthcare team, and worries about external threats and change, means that anxiety levels within individuals and the team can be overwhelming. At this point, *primitive defence mechanisms* are likely to be triggered and an understanding of these concepts can be helpful in understanding the behaviour of both the individual and the group. Like the psychological defence mechanisms described in the previous chapter, primitive defence mechanisms process anxiety but, because of the nature and degree of anxiety, characteristically distort reality and therefore amplify dysfunction.

The concept of such mental defence mechanisms sheds light on how individuals protect themselves from extreme anxiety by *denial* and un-conscious attempts to rid themselves of the feeling. An important premise is that highly disturbing emotions and thoughts – those that are so anxiety-provoking that they cannot be thought about and put into words – spill over into other people. The concept provides a model for understanding the unconscious transactions between people, how feelings are communicated when they are outside conscious awareness. It can help us think about how disturbed feelings and the cognitions that go with them can spread in teams, almost like an infection. Just as primitive defences, when they are firmly established in an individual, affect functioning and distort the identity and relationships of the person concerned, so it is in teams and wider organisations when primitive defences have become the main mode of processing emotion.

This perspective helps explain some of the processes at work in extreme situations such as Abu Ghraib and the abuse scandals in children's homes and asylums. It also throws light on the more everyday dynamics in healthcare teams overloaded with anxiety. Such understanding takes us on from the psychology experiments described earlier, which demonstrated how cruelly and unkindly many ordinary people will behave in specifically manipulated group circumstances, to a growing knowledge of what is going on within and between people in ordinary life.

Primitive defences are thought to originate in earliest infancy, before the development of language, when the infant is totally dependent on others responding to its needs for its very survival. They recur in adult life in situations of extreme anxiety, where painful reality cannot be faced in full. For some unlucky individuals, scarred by the legacy of trauma and neglect, such mechanisms can dominate their personality and make everyday living and relating an enormous struggle, not just for themselves, but for those around them. But everyone resorts to using this type of emotional processing at times of extreme stress. By definition, the element that makes them so powerful is that people do not know what they are doing: we cannot bear to acknowledge what we face, and are consequently unaware of the processes we are using to evade it. When these defences predominate in the mental life of a team, conflicts, poor communication and distraction are amplified and the focus on the core healthcare task is severely undermined. Teams can be susceptible to debilitating conflict and poor leadership. Staff are more likely to go off sick or leave the job, and there is an increased likelihood that mistakes will be made. Inevitably, attention to patients suffers.

The power of denial

Primitive defences are all based on the process of *denial*. This is common in healthcare situations, where the reality that needs to be denied is often one involving enormous risk and survival itself. Indeed, survival sometimes depends on both individuals and the team ignoring the dreadful statistic and determinedly latching on to the small chance of hope. The line between such optimism and denial is a fine one, but an important one nevertheless. Denial is a step on from repression and involves active distortion of the truth and consequent distortion of relationships. Denial frequently involves omnipotence, grandiosity and triumphalism. Some professional groups are particularly prone to these traits and in some teams they become institutionalised – in other words, they become the norm and are unquestioned. There is evidence that this was happening in the Mid-Staffordshire Trust, which was criticised for its disregard of its high mortality statistics and where it was noted that:

in spite of the criticism[s] the Trust had received recently, there is an unfortunate tendency for some staff and management to discount these by relying on the view that there is much good practice and that the reports are unfair. (Francis, 2010, p. 16)

In another trust we know of, the low returns and negative views expressed in the annual staff survey are repeatedly blamed on the staff responsible for administering the survey. This undue acceptance of procedural explanations is a common way of denying bad news.

Another all too common pattern of behaviour driven by *denial* is where a group of staff invest all their energies into a new treatment or type of therapy, so much so that they see their identities as linked with the success or otherwise of the particular treatment. The reality of disappointing outcomes and the poor immediate effect on patients, who are in danger of being over-treated, or even wrongly treated, is ignored or rationalised away. Another pattern is the team that ignores the realities of major change in the outside world (for example a change in commissioning arrangements or the development of a new competitor), denies the threat involved and rather than consider adaptations to their service, carries on as usual – almost as if they have a divine right to exist unchanged. Both these examples are exaggerated, but the dynamics are clearly recognisable in teams both inside and outside the health service. The denial at their heart is a powerful force in interpersonal and team life.

Denial prevents healthy adaptation and distorts relationships, both within a team and between the team and the outside world, as well as, critically, with patients. Two psychoanalytic concepts, *splitting* and *projective identification*, are particularly helpful to thinking in more detail about how this happens.

The theatre of love and hate

Psychoanalysts have a particular model for understanding how infants organise their experiences as emotions and how relationships develop. This is based on the idea that very young infants feel love when all is well with them, and hate when all is not well; but, existing, as they do, totally in the present, these feelings are kept totally separate from one another. Gradually, as the brain evolves and neural pathways open up, the infant develops the capacity to remember and to think about experiences in an increasingly complex and realistic fashion. As time moves on, the young child begins to be able to contemplate the reality that the same person can make them feel love *and* hate, and cope with that ambiguity. With this maturation comes the capacity both to face and cope with distress and to maintain sufficient optimism to move on.

For some people, however, and for everyone at times of extreme anxiety, memories and experiences are 'unthinkable', too full of horror and fear to be borne in mind. The pressure of illness or hospitalisation, or of working with needs that are hard to face, may well push an individual back on to infantile forms of *splitting* the world into 'good' and 'bad', the 'good' being idealised and the 'bad' denigrated. The effect of this splitting may be seen in relations between team members – and between patients and the team.

As an example, a patient with cancer, Sally, puts all her hope into complementary therapies while being negative about and uncooperative with the treatment the specialist at the hospital is offering. Clues that her response is driven by an unconscious process rather than thoughtful opinion are her vehemence and inflexibility. The consultant, for example, tries to discuss the possibility of using acupuncture for pain relief, but Sally dismisses this straightaway in the same manner that she has dismissed other suggestions. Her behaviour is driven by her extreme need to keep the 'good' and 'bad' separate in her mind. In this way, she can invest hope, uncontaminated by doubts, in the alternative therapist, while blaming the consultant for her deteriorating health. Imagine the potential effects on the team dynamic if Sally splits instead between nurses and doctors, or projects all her contempt onto one nurse while idealising the others (a particular form of group splitting known as *scapegoating*) or becomes fixed on the idea that the surgical team can do nothing wrong while the oncology team can do nothing right.

Most people have a tendency to conform to expectations (if someone believes strongly you are clumsy, you are more likely to be clumsy in their presence) and the unconscious is good at finding hooks in others on which to project unwanted feelings. Sometimes this process can exploit and perpetuate racist or gender stereotypes; sometimes it will hook on to existing personality traits; and sometimes there will be little to hook it on, and the projected feelings will sit rather oddly with the recipient.

Often, such projections can be so powerful that the recipients actually experience and identify with the feelings as if they were their own, through the process described in psychoanalysis as *projective identification*. Remember that both parties are unconscious of this dynamic and the feelings are projected in the first place only because the original person was unable to face them. It is as if the unwanted feelings are being pushed into the other person. The recipients of projective identification, experiencing the feelings as their own, are likely to act on them. At this point, things become even more complicated and difficult to disentangle, as staff members start acting on feelings of, say, incompetence, depression or anger that do not fully belong to them in the first place. It is not, of course, only the patient whose anxiety levels are so high as to provoke these processes. Individual members of staff, or groups of staff, may unconsciously (or part consciously) resort to the splitting and displacement of inconvenient or threatening realities onto colleagues within a team, or in another team.

In teams where these processes, and those indicated by Bion (see above), are at work – in all teams, some of the time – individual and collective feeling and behaviour are profoundly influenced. Where leaders and team members lack a 'mental model' of what is at work in groups, and are unable to pay attention to how the team as a whole and its members are behaving, the team is vulnerable to dysfunction and distortion of its relationships and work. Where the wider organisation is characterised by extreme forms of these processes, individual teams are more vulnerable to them.

Team resilience

From this point of view, it seems right that the recommendations in the report of the inquiry into the Mid-Staffordshire Trust mainly addressed failures in the system, rather than individual staff at the front line (Francis, 2010, pp. 398–418). Interestingly, though, it seems that there were areas of good practice within Stafford described in some of the accounts given by patients and their representatives. One contrasted the 'excellent' care on the coronary care unit with that on some of the wards, which should have brought 'shame to the nurses' uniform'; another comparing the care on ward 6 with that on ward 7, likened them to two 'different lands' (p. 159). It would seem that even within a dysfunctional umbrella organisation, there are opportunities to create islands of good team working, where attention to the needs of the patients is paramount. Research into team functioning demonstrates that thoughtful, well-managed teamwork can 'buffer' the effects of a wider dysfunctional organisation (Borrill *et al*, 2000).

Unfortunately, healthcare teams in the UK are not highly evolved in their *functioning as teams*. The quality of meetings is often poor and team objectives unclear (Borrill *et al*, 2000). Health service teams tend to be large, much larger than the ideal of six to ten that is known to promote a sense of cohesiveness and belonging, good communication and participation in decision-making (Firth-Cozens & Cornwell, 2009, p. 7). They also tend to have unclear boundaries and sometimes conflicting objectives, with different professions approaching the task from different perspectives and tensions sometimes arising between professional and organisational hierarchies. In addition, many staff are on rapid training rotations or can be moved without consultation to cover shortages in other teams. One unwanted effect of the European Working Time Directive (which set a legal maximum shift length and working week) has been the breakdown of close-knit medical 'firms', and patients have consequently complained that they see a series of junior doctors and do not know the name of their consultant. In fact, many healthcare staff, particularly senior staff, have a peripatetic role and belong in many different teams, or, as a recent paper has described them, *pseudo-teams* (Firth-Cozens & Cornwell, 2009, p. 7).

Healthy teamwork

The perspectives of social and evolutionary psychology and psychoanalysis suggest that well-managed teamwork involves the ability to contain and manage: anxiety and denial; passivity, neediness and conformism; aggression, conflict and acquisitiveness. Effective teamwork manages to minimise the playing out of those 'team dramas' that undermine people's sense of themselves and instead enables them to connect with their goodwill, capability and responsibilities.

Research clearly establishes the importance of well-functioning healthcare teams, and Borrill *et al* (2000) even established a link between the proportion of staff working in teams in a particular hospital and patient mortality – where more employees work in teams, the death rate is lower. The same authors found those working in teams had better mental health than those working in looser groups or individually and that well-functioning teams have better retention and lower turnover rates. The quality of team working is related to effectiveness in terms of clearer team objectives, better peer support, a higher level of participation by team members, greater commitment to quality and more support for innovation.

A well-established 'team' tradition within the field of mental health concerns the therapeutic environment or *milieu*. Here, healthy functioning of the staff team is seen as an essential therapeutic agent of change. Alongside and supporting this recognition that the social environment is a key aspect of treatment, conceptual and technical ways of measuring the therapeutic environment have developed, through instruments such as the Ward Atmosphere Scale (Timko & Moos, 2004). Such instruments can be used to describe and compare different types of treatment setting and to evaluate different components of the social climate and which aspects of a therapeutic programme are most likely to facilitate good outcomes. This type of action research allows an ongoing study of therapeutic environments, with everybody being involved as both an object and an agent of enquiry. The findings, implications and indeed some of the research techniques could usefully be extended beyond the field of mental health.

More generally, healthcare staff all have irreducible emotional needs that will be stirred by their work. It can be helpful to think of these needs in terms of processes of emotional development. We are all helped by a sequence of experiences to grow into people well enough adjusted in the first place and then to cope with and grow from the emotional demands that being ill or working in healthcare throws up later in life. In a paper on developmental dynamics for staff groups, Rex Haigh, a group analyst, has used this model to describe the needs of staff in healthcare settings (Haigh, 2004),

Table 5.1 Five qualities of a therapeutic environment, presented as a developmental sequence

Quality	Expression in a therapeutic environment
Attachment	A culture of belonging, in which attention is given to joining and leaving, and staff are encouraged to feel part of things
Containment	A culture of safety, in which there is a secure organisational structure and staff feel supported, looked after and cared about within the team
Communication	A culture of openness, in which difficulties and conflict can be voiced, and staff have a reflective, questioning attitude to the work
Involvement	A 'living–learning' culture, in which team members appreciate each other's contributions and have a sense that their work and perspective are valued
Agency	A culture of empowerment, in which all members of the team have a say in the running of the place and play a part in decision-making

From Haigh (2004, p. 120).

summarised in Table 5.1. Most important is the need for attachment, a sense of belonging, a fundamental requirement for establishing the relationship to one's work, on which safe and effective practice must be based. Sadly, many healthcare teams are not well structured to fulfil these needs, with some exceptions, especially in mental health, general practice and hospice work. Haigh's model, however, by focusing on underlying principles rather than prescriptive formulae, provides a framework that we can all use to reflect on and contribute to improving the social climate in the team.

Staff support groups

One way to facilitate the emotional work of teams is to set up supportive groups for staff. There are many forms this can take, from *case discussion groups* to less structured *reflective practice groups*. The regular support of a group of colleagues who face similar situations can help staff to speak out about traumatic and difficult encounters and dilemmas. As with any type of group experience, participants benefit from the support and feedback from other members of the group and one outcome of such groups should be a general increase in affiliative behaviour between team members – not just during the group sessions. Staff handovers and other staff meetings can also present opportunities for support, although this is not the same as having a regular, protected forum where psychological work is the focus.

Unfortunately, staff support groups are rare outside mental health and hospice settings; even in mental health settings, they are not the rule, despite evidence that they are helpful (Hartley & Kennard, 2009). *Balint groups* were introduced for general practitioners (GPs) in the UK in the 1940s and modified forms of such groups continue to have a place in the training of GPs and psychiatrists. As well as providing a forum where the *relationship* with patients is the focus, they challenge the isolated stoicism that is so often a characteristic of medical practice.

In the USA, multidisciplinary *Schwarz Center rounds* started up in 1997 and are now held in over 186 sites across the country. They are held for 1 hour each month – hardly a huge investment. They are designed to enhance relationships and communication among members of multidisciplinary teams and to create supportive environments in which all can learn from each other. Results of initial evaluations are positive (Lown & Manning, 2010) and the King's Fund started a pilot in two sites in the UK in 2010. Most attendees, in retrospective surveys, report an increased likelihood of attending to psychosocial and emotional aspects of care and an enhanced belief in the importance of empathy. There also seems to be a significant decrease in perceived stress and improvements in their ability to cope with the psychosocial demands of care. Better teamwork is reported, including heightened appreciation of the roles and contribution of colleagues and a sense of being less alone and better supported. The majority found the rounds had 'provided a touchstone', that is, reminded them why they entered their profession; they had strengthened relationships with colleagues and patients and counteracted the pressure to approach patient care as a business. This is of interest, given some evidence that the altruism in doctors and nurses at the start of their training has a tendency to wane (Maben *et al*, 2007).

Another important finding, in keeping with the virtuous circle outlined in this book, was that hospitals which hosted Schwartz Center rounds reported a positive change in the institutional culture and a greater focus on patient-centred policy and initiatives. The question really should be why all staff are not involved in some sort of support group where they can process some of the more difficult experiences and feelings that the work brings up.

Making the team dynamic a priority

This chapter has brought together strands of thinking from diverse theoretical backgrounds in an attempt to throw light on the reasons why people behave as they do – often irrationally and destructively – when they are part of a group, in this case, a healthcare team. There is little doubt that pressures on teams of staff in the NHS continue to increase. It cannot be assumed that even generally kind and sensible people will behave well when they are part of a team coping badly under pressure. Indeed, there is a great deal of evidence that many of us have the potential to be unthinkingly neglectful and even abusive.

In general, the NHS gives little thought to group dynamics and how to get the best out of its teams. Too often, structure and culture impede rather than enable good team working. Rare tokenistic gestures such as training events and team 'away days' are not usually followed through and are often undermined by management imperatives that have not considered the effects on the team dynamic. This throws up particular issues for an institution where the primary task is to provide humane care 'at times of most basic human need, when care and compassion are what matter most' (Department of Health, 2009). The emotional work of healthcare teams deserves to be prioritised.

The qualities, understanding and skills of staff in leadership roles are vital factors to the health of teams. Many people have the self-awareness, compassion and qualities to help teams manage their experiences and maintain a compassionate and committed focus on patient need. Many people responsible for leadership in teams and organisations have found it helpful to explore group dynamics more directly. They have committed time to develop their understanding of how groups work and to consider the implications for how they manage themselves in groups and in their roles as leaders. Learning events covering experiential group relations have been held for decades, with two main approaches involved: the group analytic approach (see http://groupanalyticsociety.co.uk) and the Bion-inspired tradition (see http://www.tavinstitute.org).

Beyond the team

A healthy team supports its individual members in the challenges of self-awareness and self-management required to maintain attentive, kind practice and to work together in the service of the patient. Just as the individual is open to helpful or unhelpful influences from the team, the team itself is constantly working within a wider system. That system requires collaboration with other teams and attention to organisational issues and processes. This, too, involves attention to how anxiety is managed, to what is being played out in relationships, how the system is organised and the values that direct it.

References

Asch, S. E. (1951) Effects of group pressure upon the modification and distortion of judgment. In *Groups, Leadership and Men* (ed. H. Guetzkow), pp. 177–190. Carnegie Press.

Bion, W. R. (1961) *Experiences in Groups*. Tavistock.

Blass, T. (ed.) (2000) *Obedience to Authority: Current Perspectives on the Milgram Paradigm*. Lawrence Erlbaum Associates.

Bond, R. & Smith, P. (1996) Culture and conformity: a meta-analysis of studies using Asch's (1952b, 1956) line judgement task. *Psychological Bulletin*, **119**, 111–137.

Borrill, C., West, M., Shapiro, D., et al (2000) Team working and effectiveness in healthcare. *British Journal of Health Care Management*, **6**, 364–371.

Department of Health (2009) *The NHS Constitution for England: The NHS Belongs To Us All*. HMSO.

Firth-Cozens, J. & Cornwell, J. (2009) *The Point of Care. Enabling Compassionate Care in Acute Hospital Settings.* King's Fund.

Francis, R. (2010) *The Independent Inquiry into Care Provided by Mid-Staffordshire NHS Foundation Trust, January 2005–March 2009.* HMSO.

Gilbert, P. (2009) *The Compassionate Mind.* Constable and Robinson.

Haigh, R. (2004) The quintessence of an effective team: some developmental dynamics for staff groups. In *From Toxic Institutions to Therapeutic Environments* (ed. P. Campling & R. Haigh), pp. 119–130. Royal College of Psychiatrists.

Haney, C., Bank, W. C. & Zimbardo, P. G. (1973) Interpersonal dynamics in a simulated prison. *International Journal of Criminology and Penology*, 1, 69–97.

Hartley, P. & Kennard, D. (2009) *Staff Support Groups in the Helping Professions. Principles, Practice and Pitfalls.* Routledge.

Lown, B. A. & Manning, C. F. (2010) The Schwartz Center rounds: evaluation of an interdisciplinary approach to enhancing patient-centred communication, treatment and provider support. *Academic Medicine*, 85, 1073–1081.

Maben, J., Latter, S. & Macleod Clark, J. (2007) The sustainability of ideals, values and the nursing mandate: evidence from a longitudinal qualitative study. *Nursing Inquiry*, 14, 99–111.

Milgram, S. (1963) Behavioural study of obedience. *Journal of Abnormal and Social Psychology*, 67, 371–378.

Reicher, S. & Haslam, S. (2006) Rethinking the psychology of tyranny: the BBC Prison Study. *British Journal of Social Psychology*, 45, 1–40.

Timko, C. & Moos, R. H. (2004) Measuring the therapeutic environment. In *From Toxic Institutions to Therapeutic Environments* (ed. P. Campling & R. Haigh), pp. 143–156. Royal College of Psychiatrists.

CHAPTER 6

Cooperation and fragmentation

The only thing that will redeem mankind is cooperation. (Bertrand Russell)

Fragmented systems

The team is a vital medium in which to nourish attentive and compassionate work with patients. The way a team manages anxiety, work pressures, interpersonal relationships and its tasks can bring the best out in its members and create a buffer against organisational processes that might otherwise tend to undermine patient-centred care. But teams are not 'islands', and this chapter shifts to focus on the wider system. The increasingly sophisticated specialist expertise and technologies that have developed, and the complexity of organisational and management systems typically involved in a patient's journey, mean that the relationships between teams are as important as the relationships within the team. For example, a cancer patient may need a combination of primary care, general medicine, surgery, radiotherapy, radiology, pathology and hospice care. The overall quality of cancer care this patient receives will depend not on the presence of a brilliant single health professional or team but on each professional interacting well with all the other involved elements of the system.

It is not uncommon to hear of patients being sent from one end of the hospital to the other, turning up for investigations at departments that have never heard of them, waiting for hours while their notes are tracked down, having to recount their story over and over again. Experiences like this are not just inconvenient: they break down patients' trust and the capacity of the system to attend to their needs. Patients will not feel kindly treated if their experience is fragmented and if there is no continuity of relationship. If communication between teams is inadequate, staff will not have the personal and detailed information about the patient that makes kindness so much easier. Poor communication can underpin poor care, neglect and error. Many reports into tragedies involving people with a mental illness or in child protection have highlighted discontinuity and breakdowns in communication, with a consequent loss of a whole view of patients and of a real personal connection with them (Ritchie, 1994; Laming, 2003). In a recent report by the National Confidential Enquiry into Patient Outcomes and Death (NCEPOD), poor communication between and within teams was identified as an important factor in 13.5% of the deaths studied. The authors observed that:

Change in hospital team structure over recent years has seen individual clinicians become transient acquaintances during a patient's illness rather than having any continuity of care. (NCEPOD, 2009, p. 7)

Teams must, then, find ways of working together and sharing information. This task is often reduced to one of procedures and information systems, but it is at least as important to see it as dependent on relationships within and between teams. The question is how to strengthen a continuous attentive and compassionate link with the patient that inspires good communication and collaboration. The way a team relates to the wider system and the ways in which relationships and collaboration between teams are organised powerfully influence both the capacity of staff to work kindly with the patient and the patient's experience of the system. If these issues are appropriately addressed, kindness in practice can be encouraged and liberated, but all approaches can fail unless implementation is informed by consideration of how the system influences teams and individuals.

Team boundaries

A helpful way of looking at team behaviour in systems is by considering how a team manages its *boundaries*. These include membership, space, time, task and role. How a team manages its boundaries influences how well it is able to communicate and cooperate with other teams and their representatives. Thinking about such boundary management can be helped by four categories of question:

- How *open* is the team to welcoming and including 'outsiders' in work with the patient, and ready to think about their perspective and concerns?
- How flexible is the team about *where* it operates – where it will meet others, where it will deliver its service?
- How flexible is the team about *when* it does its work – opening hours, sessions and clinics, waiting lists and duty systems, and so on?
- How rigid or flexible is the team about what its *task* should be and about the roles it is ready to take on in partnership with others to meet patient need?

In each case there is a pull between being too 'tight' and too 'loose' in managing the boundary. Too tight, and the team will be hard to work with, inaccessible and rigid, pursuing its own agenda instead of working to a collective plan. Too loose, and the team will be ill-equipped to focus on its task and maintain quality and dependability in its work. Each boundary should be established through a balance of the team's needs to focus on its own tasks and its ability to work flexibly with others *in the service of the patient*. The better this balance is in all the teams in a wider system, the more ready and able their members will be to work together across team boundaries. Communication, information sharing and joint consideration of the patient will be facilitated the more staff feel able to work together across these boundaries. The more staff are able to build relationships, the less obscured and fragmented the picture of the patient in the minds of the staff will be, and the patient's sense of being met and held in mind as a person will be reinforced.

Boundary management is not a simple matter of procedure and operational policy. Feelings can be transferred across a boundary in both directions. The way a team manages its relationships with others can be influenced by what is happening inside the team. Anxiety, if not faced and managed maturely, can spill over into the way the team relates to the world outside. This anxiety might be aroused by inter-professional conflicts in the team, by difficult responsibilities for tasks, performance or people. Feelings belonging within the team can be transferred to people outside – especially managers, referrers and other colleagues – who can then begin to be seen as persecutory, uncooperative, withholding or incompetent. Even where a team needs to protect itself from genuinely unhealthy realities outside, this kind of externalised aggression or defensiveness is unhelpful. The less cooperative and effectively responsive a team is in a wider system, the more likely the patient is to suffer from discontinuity and errors. The more relationships are coloured by defence mechanisms (discussed in the previous chapter), the less the patient's reality will be attended to. The culture of a team and, in particular, the nature and intensity of the defence mechanisms at work will determine how the team manages its boundaries (Zagier Roberts, 1994).

The wider care system is made up of teams, departments and organisations, all of which may manage their own boundaries well or badly, who may bring openness and cooperation or negative, self-protective, attitudes and feelings to partnership work. The consequent 'landscape' through which staff – and the patient – must move involves encounters with these boundaries. How they experience this landscape profoundly affects the emotional climate, and the conditions for kindness.

Narrowing down the primary task

Where boundary management in teams within a wider system is too much infected by defensiveness, that system can become seriously dysfunctional. At the very least, there is no collective agreement about and alignment with what should be the primary task – *bringing all of the required resources from across the system kindly together to help the patient*. At the worst, we get the ugly sight of teams accusing each other of 'dumping' patients on them, or otherwise denigrating each other, with a consequent resentful colouring of relationships with patients.

The problem of embattled teams fragmenting the system of care needed by the patient can be found in all aspects of healthcare. But it seems to be at its worst when the patient has a condition that is chronic rather than acute, where interventions are low on technology, reliant on people and mainly provided in the community – elderly patients with dementia being an obvious example. Staff teams working in such areas will usually acknowledge that needs are high and that resources are far from adequate. This can lead to a tendency for teams to manage their own part within the system by narrowing the definition of their primary task. They tell themselves they are doing – or being asked to do – much more than is expected, and at the same time project their sense of inadequacy onto other teams. Management of task boundaries is infected by defence mechanisms.

A classic example from psychiatry is that of the patient who suffers from schizophrenia and also misuses illegal drugs. There is a general sense that such patients pose complex clinical management problems that tend to overwhelm the available resources and therapeutic skills. Staff on acute general psychiatry wards often tell themselves their 'task' is to work with people who are mentally ill, so having to care for people with drug problems is going over and above what they are there to do. The drug teams usually define their primary task as working with drug users, the priority depending on the class of drug as defined by the Home Office. In other words, both teams are sure they are doing more than they should for people with the dual diagnosis, and they tend to blame the other team for doing a lot less than they should. Their definitions of the primary task are a way of keeping guilt and a sense of failure at bay.

Of course, there are probably areas of the country where care for those with a dual diagnosis is exemplary. In general, however, despite various policy initiatives, unhelpful splitting of the task between teams with different backgrounds and perspectives tends to be difficult to change. Most healthcare staff will be able to relate to similar situations and recognise such stock phrases as 'we are not really supposed to...', 'it's not really our responsibility...', 'we're not set up to deal with incontinence...', 'I wasn't trained to do this...'.

In his book, *Managing Vulnerability*, Tim Dartington, a researcher and consultant in health and social care, previously of the Tavistock Institute of Human Relations in London, explores this phenomenon, with a particular focus on the split between health and social services in the care of the elderly. He is interested in why the split seems so intractable and notes:

there appears to be an unconscious wish to act out the insolubility of an intractable problem – that people get older and weaker – by taking sides, even when this becomes dysfunctional. (Dartington, 2010, p. 93)

He sees the 'defining down' of the task as in the examples above as a symptom of stress, increasingly out of touch with reality (p. 96). In the face of overwhelming vulnerability and helplessness in the patients they are caring for, teams like to see themselves as in control of their working environment and end up behaving as if there are no other stakeholders and no wider system within which to negotiate compromises.

The normative task (what we ought to do) is defined down, as within a closed system, as if it is not subject to vagaries of the environment. The existential task (what we think we are doing) is opened out as if the system is being flooded by the environment. In the perception of those that live and work in them, care systems are inadequate to meet the challenges that face them, but it is not their fault. (p. 97)

It is the way processes like this colour the way teams manage their boundaries that requires attention if the patient as a person is to find real recognition and cooperative compassion in the care system. To create the conditions for such healthy joint work requires work at individual team level, to develop a mature culture internally and to attend constructively to boundaries. The way the wider care system is structured, organised and led, and the contracts and specifications that shape it, are also important. Attending to these 'business' factors can create conditions within which healthier relationships are more likely, but without attention to team and system dynamics and their effects on boundaries, they will be of limited effectiveness, and may even do real damage to compassionate care.

Pulled in all directions

At their worst, organisational factors can cause serious fragmentation of teamwork and of relationships between teams. One of our parents was recently assessed for a knee replacement. On asking how long she should expect to stay in hospital after the operation, she received a surprisingly complicated answer. If she lived within the area covered by the city primary care trust (PCT) she would be discharged when she was felt to be clinically ready; if she lived within the area covered by the county PCT, she would be discharged after 2 days. Presumably the county PCT had commissioned a community-based service by diverting some of the funding from the acute hospital trust. The rights and wrongs of these two different systems are not the issue here, but the story illustrates how such factors can complicate tasks and relationships. Two different regimes were being applied in the same ward. The work for the staff caring for 'county' patients was significantly different from their care for 'city' patients. The pace of work, the relationship with the patient, even the core task, with each group was different. With county patients, from return from surgery, the primary task was preparing them for discharge; with city patients, it was getting them well enough to go home. As a result, the ward team were vulnerable. Staff were being asked to look through two very different, very influential lenses. Their consideration of the patient in each category was different, so that attunement to the patient's needs, judgements about care, communication and decision-making between staff members were liable to confusion or even conflict. However committed and professional the staff were, their quality of attention, their focus and priorities would inevitably have been affected.

The fragmentation of the ward team's task would have gone further. Managing relationships and work with two kinds of community services would be complicated. Boundaries of time, place and task would have been different, with different professional and emotional agendas. Ward staff would have been looking for different things from their county colleagues than they would from city colleagues. In the case of the county, the hospital team would have been negotiating work more rapidly, with higher levels of need and higher levels of risk involved. There would have been a greater need to communicate well with the primary and community healthcare teams and to educate the patients' 'carers' (meaning family or friends) to take on some of the tasks that the ward staff would be doing for city patients. Given the higher levels of need being managed in the community, hospital specialists would need – and would want – to influence the 'county' model and the nature and quality of post-operative care in the community received by their patients.

As a result of there being two systems, orthopaedic surgeons, physio- and occupational therapists and nurses in the hospital would need to be involved in developing and working within two different care pathways, with different clinical protocols, audit approaches and training. The pressure on time, and the potential for confusion of paperwork, let alone the more serious issues relating to clarity of task, raise serious concerns.

In fact, it is not unusual for acute hospital services to have to work within different agreements with various commissioners and community services. As patients exercise choice of hospital, GPs and community health services will be faced increasingly with similar complications – different hospitals will have different ways of operating, with different expectations from local services. Our orthopaedic example demonstrates the power of fragmented commissioning and contracting arrangements to disrupt and complicate teamwork and inter-team relationships. There are many other examples of organisational issues creating such dynamics. Working with different local authority eligibility and charging regimes for social care or with variations in community health and/or primary care models can all complicate and confuse. Such organisational factors can add an extra dimension to boundary management and relationships within a healthcare system. They also affect the experience of patients. In the example, people in neighbouring beds were, to varying extents, aware of the different regimes and mind-sets, and were often uncertain and anxious as a result. Some patients heard staff refer to them as 'breachers' (of the discharge target), with predictable effects on their morale.

In this example, the application of contracts and working practices, and the effect on the emotional life of staff and patients, work directly against the actualisation of kindness. They seriously disrupt the 'virtuous circle' outlined in Chapter 3.

Promoting collaborative working

The issue of collaborative working is all the more significant when people are being cared for in the community. Here, typically, several agencies, and staff from different parts of each agency, will be involved. The need to bring continuity and integration to this cross-boundary collaboration, and the variety of journeys which patients must take through services, have been recognised and addressed from a number of perspectives in health policy and service development. Attempts have been made to bring consistency and clarity through two main approaches: *structural integration*, with the creation of formal inter-agency teams; and *care pathway* development within networks across agencies.

Structural integration

Structural integration – creating inter-agency teams, or even whole services – has been employed to try to bring together the work of a range of agencies and professions to treat the patient as a whole person. These developments have been core parts of strategy in mental health and, to a lesser extent, intellectual disabilities and older people's services. In such models the 'integration' may be between health and social care staff, acute and community healthcare staff, or representatives of different disciplines. At their best, integrated teams can make a big difference, promoting much more patient-centred and collaborative practice. Frequently, though, such work has focused on form rather than function, on bureaucracy and governance rather than on the benefits for the patient. Sitting various professions together is only part of the solution. The degree to which such integration has improved collaboration and communication between staff has sometimes been undermined by a failure to recognise the way diffuse professional, organisational and performance accountabilities continue to hamper joint work. Staff have genuinely to be – and feel – free and available to work together. They need professional support, organisational and infor- mation systems, and an accountability framework that enable this.

It is surprising how common it is for even integrated teams to be bedevilled by dysfunctional information systems – for the wider system it is the rule, rather than the exception. Staff from different agencies, whether configured into integrated teams or not, often use incompatible and different systems – which cannot communicate with each other, exclude some staff from access, and which record and recognise the patient in different ways. Attempts to create comprehensive, global systems across the NHS have not borne fruit. Primary care teams continue to use their own systems, which are different from those in community services, whose systems are different from those of mental health services, and so on. It is easy to imagine how this could prejudice the care of, say, an older person with diabetes, a fractured femur and memory problems.

Failure to develop effective confidentiality and access protocols seriously undermines integrated work, especially between health and local authority staff. Instead of being a dependable and integrated resource for bearing patients in mind and communicating about them, information technology becomes a frustration, a 'beast' that needs feeding and coping with. Valuable time and emotional energy are diverted from the patient to compensate for problems with information systems, with duplication of records and reports, uncertainty and sometimes dangerous gaps in knowledge.

Bringing together some parts of the system in joint teams has often involved losing sight of the fact that there are *always* services the patient needs that lie outside the circle of 'integration'. While integration can be effective, it can also obscure the need to continue to attend to the relationships between professions and to the boundaries between teams that have such a strong influence on the ability of all staff involved collectively to engage sensitively with the patient as a person. Various approaches to organising and managing roles and relationships across disparate systems of care have been introduced. Most are based on the aim of putting the patient at the centre of a smoothly operating, well-organised system. When they work well, they can support staff to work with the kinds of attentiveness and attunement involved in the application of kindness. This is not, though, inevitable.

Care pathways

Achieving healthcare boundary management involves promoting the attitudes, confidence and space for staff to become effective partners in wider 'virtual teams', with the patient at their centre. It is best addressed by offering teams within a wider system the chance to work out together how they might collaborate to bear the patient in mind, how they need to communicate, and what values should underpin relationships and joint work.

Commissioning for, and the organisation of, *integrated care pathways* that shape the work of *clinical networks* across several agencies can contribute to helping disparate services work together. For a particular kind of need, a care pathway may specify such elements as:
- assessment tools and processes
- clinical and therapeutic interventions and their intended outcome
- the roles and responsibilities of different professionals
- the timing and sequencing of elements of care.

The approach aims to guarantee a standard of care, based on evidence and, where relevant, legal and ethical factors. Care pathways can help both to clarify what the patient's journey through treatment will look like, and to secure effective agreement across disciplines and organisations to making it happen. They can help foster healthy and patient-focused collaboration across and between teams and services. They are most effective when the clinical dimension of the pathway is supported by clear systems and intra- and inter-organisational processes that will make care available in the way the pathway indicates.

There is a danger, though, that pathways can become mechanical, mere manuals for menu-based interventions. It is important to get the right balance between prescription and flexibility in care pathway work, to ensure that staff are genuinely able to attend and respond to patient ill-being. Too much prescription, too many checklists, and staff become mechanical in their efforts – too little, and vital services are poorly organised to respond to patient need. Staff who feel like cogs in a machine, or who are frustrated by the gap between intentions and reality, are unlikely to be able to bring kindly attention to the patient.

Another challenge is to make pathway development comprehensive and genuinely inclusive. Pathways are, of course, much easier to design and implement where there is a clear and boundaried process – the journey into hospital and through cardiac surgery, for example – and where there is a relatively boundaried group of staff involved. Unsurprisingly, then, much pathway development has been undertaken in specific care settings rather than from a 'whole system' perspective. Pathways that indicate what will be offered to patients as they 'travel through' a particular ward, team or service, or that embody agreements only about roles and systems in one organisation are common. The real 'journey' for the patient often requires the cooperation of more than one organisation, and the coordination of staff from several teams, with their own duty and referral systems, waiting lists, working hours and so on. Effective communication and cooperation across this wider system are essential if there is to be real focus on promoting patient well-being.

There is often a question over whom the pathway is actually for. Too often, it specifies *a journey for the patient into and through* a series of services or interventions. Such an approach may be appropriate when there is the need for a clear and relatively short-term process of assessment, diagnosis and intervention, and a predictable journey of recovery. However, with longer-term conditions, and especially severe mental health difficulties or age-related infirmity, what is more important is *how services will organise themselves, separately and together, to get care to the patient.*

The question of whose pathway it is can be raised in rather sad ways. In our recent visit to the orthopaedic surgical ward, we found an extensive graphic display of a 'continence pathway' for nurses on the walls of the public(!) entry area. Management of continence problems is vital, and there have been repeated concerns, even scandals, as to how hospitals manage them. Staff need to know, and institutions need to demonstrate to inspectors that they know, how to work with incontinence.

The patient we were visiting, though, was a very astute 80-year-old woman, a walker and a winter sea swimmer, recovering from a knee replacement operation. She languished for 2 weeks in her bed under a sticker announcing she was a 'point of care'. From her point of view, the pathway she was interested in involved a journey, avoiding infection and falls, towards increased mobility and rehabilitation at home. Nowhere was there public evidence that such a pathway existed. She received sporadic and disconnected visits from physio- and occupational therapists, but no coordinated rehabilitation plan, advice or intervention, and was discharged home with no follow-up planned or arranged, and armed only with a pitifully short advice booklet. Unsurprisingly, subsequent complications were hard for her, and made worse by the fact that she had no clear sense of the pathway she was actually travelling along, or its risks, decision points, rules and resources available.

Care pathways can encourage collaborative care, responsive to the patient as a whole person, if the following key issues are addressed:

- Ensure pathway development is built around responding to what will matter to, and improve the experience of and outcomes for, the patient, not the service(s). Build ways of gathering patient experience into the formal processes of the pathway, rather than leaving them to separate 'user consultation' processes.
- Map out which organisations to include in pathway development on the basis of this picture of the patient's situation and needs.
- Involve staff – and, wherever appropriate, patients – at all levels across the system in networks that reflect current joint work and evidence and best practice.
- Help these networks to develop and own their local pathway.
- Facilitate agreement about the values, ground rules and behaviours expected of participating teams and services as they work with the patient and together, and make such things *formal* parts of the pathway.
- Identify and secure the agreements required at organisational level to enable access to personnel, resources and skills at the times and in the circumstances indicated by the pathway.
- Support networks across organisational boundaries to review and address how they are working together. Ensure that such review includes patient experience *and* the experience of collaboration across boundaries. Sustain networks' attention to continuous improvement.
- Ensure that management teams are focused on delivering services 'into' the agreed pathways, and that workforce planning, training and management are driven by their needs. Too often such teams can be collections of fragmented 'departments' and their particular interests.
- Ensure that commissioning is focused on delivering the pathway, not on securing fragmented bundles of activity undertaken by disconnected contract-holding organisations.

Clinical networks

Care pathways can be used as ways of organising the efforts of staff across disciplines, departments and agencies. The networks of staff involved in delivering the care involved can be informal or formally recognised and managed, and sometimes commissioned and funded directly. The pathway is then delivered by the clinical network. The *managed clinical network* (MCN) approach has been adopted in a number of areas, starting in Scotland with cancer care (Scottish Office, 1999; Kunkler, 2002).

There are obvious benefits to planning and managing systems of care in this way, but great care and some circumspection are required if truly effective networks are to be established. There is a substantial tension between a predominant culture in which individual, hierarchical organis-ations ply their trades, and a model involving *horizontal collaboration*, pooled resources and risks. A number of recent papers offer a critique of MCNs using comparisons or case histories of particular networks to identify what is and is not effective and sustainable (e.g. Hamilton *et al*, 2005; Green *et al*, 2009). There is growing evidence that some MCNs have not lived up to expectations and have wasted resources – particularly the time, energy and enthusiasm of staff and patients, who have been left disappointed and cynical.

The challenges identified by MCNs clarify the inherent problems in the system that any attempt to work collaboratively across team and organisation boundaries has to transcend. Such challenges include those in the following list, adapted from Royal College of Paediatrics and Child Health (2006):

- the sheer complexity of provision
- varying structures which do not map onto one another
- incompatible systems and policies across agencies (e.g. information technology systems, inspection methods, commonly used terminology)
- contrary policy directions
- different approaches to quality improvement
- concern about information-sharing across agencies
- lack of commissioning capacity
- fragmented commissioning practice
- variable quality of commissioning
- policies such as payment by results and practice-based commissioning
- a shortage of high-quality information on which to base decisions
- organisational inertia, bureaucracy and unwillingness to change
- preoccupation in organisations with challenges such as meeting the demands of the European Working Time Directive, targets and existing overspends
- imbalance of power between consumers and providers.

There is no single model for an optimal network and many of the papers describe the advantages and disadvantages of different models and emphasise the creative tension, constant balancing act and need to compromise. A tension repeatedly described in the literature is around how much an MCN exercises direct authority, takes on a regulatory function or introduces a hierarchical element to the structure. While the advantages of moving in this direction in terms of ensuring a rapid, coordinated response to a problem are clear, MCNs are often poor in gaining support and commitment from network professionals and can end up stifling motivation and creativity.

A number of MCNs are described as having lost touch with their original aspirations, under the pressure of the target culture (Addicott *et al*, 2007). Clearly, the task of managing and implementing service improvement across a number of organisations is problematic. There are examples of MCNs, which, while finding it relatively easy to reach consensus on objectives and priorities, have found it difficult to implement service improvement. While it is tempting to establish operational procedures through formalised contracts and agreements, imposing tight regulation from the top risks disharmony and demotivation. A key lesson is the need actively to engage respected professionals within networks, who can then promote the network to their peers.

Not surprisingly, the literature identifies good leadership as a consistent distinguishing factor between MCNs that were seen as successful and those that were not. With good leadership, it is possible to negotiate for – rather than impose – a degree of central management direction because members and member organisations are persuaded of the benefits.

MCNs can bring together staff across organisational boundaries to work cooperatively, centring their combined work on patient need, motivated by a common vision and sense of community. When this happens, the conditions for kindness are strengthened. The evidence is, though, that intensive attention to the factors working against such collaboration is required if the potential benefits of MCNs are to be realised.

Putting the patient at the centre

These approaches are, of course, focused on what services can do to bring coherence and continuity to the care of patients. Another approach has been to consider how to put power in the hands of the patient. Initially, this policy approach involved 'choice' – the guarantee that patients will be able to select where they receive secondary care – and there have been commitments made to extending this right to the choice of primary care. Associated with this trend in policy has been the concept, first introduced in social care policy, of 'personalisation', which may bring control to the patient over a budget for a 'package' of healthcare (Department of Health, 2010). These initiatives may well bring more power to the patient – at least those who want it (many do not) and are in any condition to exercise it (many have limited capability to take it up). But there is no evidence that it will guarantee better, or kinder, care.

Choosing care based on inspection reports would have exposed many to hospital infection and conditions ranging from poor to appalling in many 'flagship trusts'. Choice over how to spend resources, over types or packages of care, or over the provider of these services is clearly of value to some. Buying care patients have 'designed for themselves' with a personalised budget, if the bureaucracy involved is manageable, may open up the prospect of some small sense of being in charge, some power to withdraw a tiny bit of funding from an unsatisfactory provider. But increasing marginal 'consumer power' in this way is not the same as ensuring compassionate, effective care. Indeed, it can further depersonalise care by turning the process into something like a visit to a supermarket. What choice will not guarantee is the right attitudes and skills, and the right kind of collaboration, across a variety of agencies and staff: it may specify what patients want, but cannot ensure that they are recognised and understood sensitively across the system.

A more genuinely person-centred – and powerful – approach is the idea of 'care coordination'. This approach was first introduced in mental health in the 1990s and has been promoted through policies relating to long-term conditions (Department of Health, 1999). Judging from the evidence of failures of well-coordinated care for very vulnerable people in acute healthcare, there is a strong argument for considering its role in that and other settings. Many of us are well able to assert our needs and navigate through complex healthcare systems. Many of us, because of mental frailty, complex disabilities, risk or vulnerability, require varying degrees of help, from someone who knows and understands us, to assert our needs and to secure the continuity-focused care we need. Models have been introduced that recognise varying 'tiers' of coordination, ranging from self-care, through care coordinated by GPs, to coordination by specialist community health and social care practitioners. Varying levels of attention to differing degrees of vulnerability and to the complexity of care have been built into these models.

At its best, this approach suggests a personal relationship between a 'care coordinator' and a patient. Such a relationship involves understanding of and sensitivity to the patient's experience and needs, understanding of the range of care required and planned, and of what is involved for the patient in getting it. It requires the willingness and power on the part of the coordinator to hold in mind the patient as a whole person – ill-being and beyond – and actively to ensure that all elements of the system of care around them respond accordingly. Care coordination involves ensuring that the 'journey' through the care system is as smooth and as comprehensible as possible, that people listen and that important things are not overlooked or forgotten along the way. A care coordinator can support more effective and satisfying patient choice. The role can bring to life otherwise over-procedural or technical care pathways, by injecting an attentive relationship into the system. It offers a real opportunity for maintaining the human focus of healthcare.

Many staff in primary and community health services would, in principle, value this relationship with and responsibility to the patient. Unfortunately, this does not mean that care coordination has thrived. The limited time for patient contact and attention available to GPs in particular, and the workloads of specialist community staff, make real attention to such relationships difficult. High levels of bureaucracy – especially, in mental health, infused with risk aversion and associated performance management – frequently make the work unappealing. The role is often seen as 'drudge' or low-status work, or as a recipe for being landed with isolated personal responsibility for risk, for dealing with the problems of waiting lists, limited resources and professional and organisational politics. Professions often compete *not* to undertake this responsibility. It is tragic that a role that should maintain the human relationship at the heart of healthcare, with rewards for patient and healthcare worker alike, is treated and seen in these ways. How can knowing patients, being their guide, friend and supporter through anxiety and distress, being the orchestrator of the life-enhancing, sometimes life-saving, care they need not be regarded as a valuable aspect of professional identity?

Unless the true value and role of care coordination are reflected in staffing levels, a key chance genuinely to personalise healthcare will be missed. Unless the status, power and autonomy of care coordinators are strengthened, unless bureaucracy is reduced, and information systems improved, a real opportunity for kinship in action will be squandered. It is also likely that attempts to move the focus of healthcare out into the community, to reduce acute admissions (and costs) will fail unless this challenge is addressed.

What should not be overlooked is that care coordinators have, with their patients, to negotiate their way through complex systems. Simply giving them the nominal authority and responsibility to secure what a patient needs from the care system is no magic solution to the boundary problems we have noted. Frequently, care coordinators report that agreements they make with colleagues are not carried through, or that they, the care coordinators, are not kept informed appropriately. They may encounter defensive or dismissive responses from people involved in the patient's care. Making sure that all parts of the healthcare system recognise the role will help, as will giving care coordinators a voice to influence how collaboration develops across care systems. Placing the ability of teams to work well with care coordination alongside the other key factors in boundary management will help. Fundamentally, though, systems that ask individual coordinators to navigate through helpful and unhelpful, easy and challenging aspects of the 'diplomatic relations' across their boundaries owe those individuals respect, attention and emotional support. To strengthen the kindliness to the patient of the collaborative system, care coordinators deserve kindness themselves.

The divided focus of team leadership

Teams, then, are part of a wider system that functions better if relationships, and the processes that can undermine them, are addressed – and, indeed, if collaborative thinking is built into all aspects of work. The system can be commissioned and structured, with systems and roles to facilitate compassionate collaboration, but much relies on the quality of leadership. Effective leadership is vital to how well teams function in themselves and to how well they collaborate with others to focus on the needs of patients. Good leadership involves being able to manage a role on the interface between the team and the outside world, with one eye on its care task, and the other on the wider system.

A challenge here is that the increasing complexity of the healthcare system means that senior members of staff are increasingly drawn away from the care task towards establishing and sustaining a network of external relationships. While vital, this work inevitably takes them away from being the vigilant presence that is so badly needed on the front line, where often young and inexperienced staff are left to get on with addressing their task of caring for patients as best they can. Kindness is easily overwhelmed by pressures. If it is not actively sustained and modelled, it will be the first thing to go. A tension is then frequently set up between two essential tasks: the management of the system; and the leadership of the caring task. This tension requires careful attention. Great care is needed to support leaders to manage anxieties that may drive them to lose focus on either aspect of their role, or to find safety in over-involvement in one at the expense of the other.

Bureaucracy, governance and other organisational business tend, in general, to draw leaders *away* from the caring task. The average healthcare organisation places enormous pressures, driven by anxieties about money, performance, inspection and so on, on its senior staff to invest their time and energy in such work. The cost to front-line care – and to collaborative work – is rarely evaluated. It is painfully common to hear critical (and often senior) voices confronting people for not attending such business process meetings, but far rarer to hear them criticise staff for leaving their caring task. This is a situation that requires attention: priorities and use of human resources need to be reconsidered. If improved focus on patient need is the goal, the key roles for clinical leaders are within their own team, and in such collaborative clinical networks as we have discussed in relation to care pathways. Room for these roles needs to be made.

References

Addicott, R., McGivern, G. & Ferlie, E. (2007) The distortion of a managerial technique? The case of clinical networks in UK health care. *British Journal of Management*, **18**, 93–105.

Dartington, T. (2010) *Managing Vulnerability: The Underlying Dynamics of Systems of Care*. Karnac.

Department of Health (1999) *Effective Care Co-ordination in Mental Health Services*. HMSO.

Department of Health (2010) *Personalisation Through Person-Centred Planning*. HMSO.

Green, A., Pagliari, C., Cunningham, S., *et al* (2009) Do managed clinical networks improve quality of diabetes care? Evidence from a retrospective mixed methods evaluation. *Quality and Safety in Health Care*, **18**, 456–461.

Hamilton, K. E., Sullivan, F. M., Donnan, P. J., *et al* (2005) A managed clinical network for cardiac services; set up, operation and impact on patient care. *International Journal of Integrated Care*, **5**, e10.

Kunkler, I. H. (2002) Managed clinical networks: a new paradigm for clinical medicine. *Journal of the Royal College of Physicians*, **34**, 320–323.

Laming, H. (2003) *The Victoria Climbie Inquiry.* HMSO.

NCEPOD (2009) *Deaths in Acute Hospitals: Caring to the End?* National Confidential Enquiry into Patient Outcomes and Death. Available at http://www.ncepod.org.uk/2009dah.htm (last accessed March 2011).

Ritchie, J. (1994) *The Report of the Inquiry into the Care and Treatment of Christopher Clunis.* HMSO.

Royal College of Paediatrics and Child Health (2006) *A Guide to Understanding and Implementing Networks.* RCPCH. Available at http://www.rcpch.ac.uk/doc.aspx?id_Resource=1739 (last accessed March 2011).

Scottish Office (1999) *Cancer. Introduction of Managed Clinical Networks Within the NHS in Scotland.* Scottish Office.

Zagier Roberts, V. (1994) The organization of work: contributions from open systems theory. In *The Unconscious At Work* (eds A. Obholzer & V. Roberts), pp. 28–38. Brunner–Routledge.

CHAPTER 7

On the edges of kinship

The fault in aliens is that those easiest to exploit are the hardest
to assimilate
(Anonymous)

Powerful political and psychosocial processes influence the extent to which
society recognises and responds to its members as kin. There are difficult
'edges' at which goodwill and rejection compete for dominance in the
public mind. Healthcare staff are frequently working at these edges, which
complicate the 'self-overcoming' involved in any form of healthcare work
(see Chapter 4, p. 54). Sometimes the dilemma is pretty obvious – the
violent drunk haemorrhaging in an accident and emergency department
inevitably arouses conflicting responses; the heavy smoker in need of a
lung transplant confronts us with mixed feelings. The continued, often
dangerously fluctuating, needs of people with long-term conditions persist
in frustrating our instinct and wish to remove suffering and can wear us
down. Generosity, and the instinct to turn away, to deprive, even to punish,
vie for dominance in our thinking.

These 'edges of kinship' are sometimes much more complicated. They
may involve attitudes to people who come from 'outside' our geographical
and social boundary – such as migrants and asylum seekers. Just as
significantly, other such 'edges' involve the needs of people who are
objectively already part of our national 'kin' – such as people with profound
intellectual disabilities, mental health problems, the old and the dying.

Such groups can arouse inclusive, generous and compassionate responses.
They have the capacity, though, to evoke feelings of fear and the wish to
reject or deny either things about others or, at the deepest level, about
ourselves. The refugee evokes 'indigent' anxiety and competitive feelings
about possessions, security, work, identity, culture. The dying person
evokes helplessness in the healthy, and profound fears and rage about an
inescapable and frightening reality; the person with an intellectual disability,
a fear of dependency and difference; the psychotic individual, a fear of their
disturbance and of our own madness. These feelings are, of course, not

restricted to healthcare. They reflect wider social uncertainty, complexity of feelings, division and discrimination. They reflect profound anxieties about the extent of our resources, material and emotional, and where they should be invested. They confront us all with the limits to our generosity and fellow feeling.

In a mix with our more kindly and generous instincts, our ambivalent, reluctant or even hostile feelings about including 'the other' as kin find expression at a policy level, at a service level and at the level of the individual healthcare practitioner. This dynamic requires clear recognition and work to manage the danger to compassionate practice. A common feature of many of the groups at the edges of kinship is that discrimination and abuses in the healthcare of their members are frequently reported. Such occurrences result, often repetitively, in policies and programmes to address stigma, provide education and specify corrective action. There is a danger, however, that these abuses will continue if the complexity of what underpins neglect and brutality is not recognised more thoroughly.

There seem to be a number of overlapping themes which emerge when working on the edges of kinship:

- being confronted with frightening need and experience that threaten to overwhelm, arousing enormous anxiety about our capacity to respond
- difficult feelings, ranging from compassion to anger and hostility
- a profound struggle between the urge to include and exclude
- polarisation of thinking, frequently involving extremes of idealisation and denigration.

These themes operate both at the level of the staff member working with the individual patient and at the level of society addressing the challenges raised by particular categories of patients. Examples from groups clearly on the 'edge' can educate our understanding of the difficulties involved in providing healthcare 'on the edges of kinship'. They also throw light on the challenges to kind and compassionate healthcare more generally.

Overwhelming need

One colleague described the look some of her clients gave her which made her feel she was the only person left in the world who could help them. It was a look she had not previously encountered in many years working as a psychiatric social worker. This look is not unlike that of the totally dependent infant. It can induce powerful feelings of responsibility and protectiveness or, conversely, a wish to disengage in order to escape the weight of so much need.... However, there is another look which seems like that of someone returned from the dead: the haunted look of eyes that have seen unspeakable horrors, perhaps horrors that the mind can no longer remember. (Blackwell, 2005, p. 72)

Dick Blackwell, a psychotherapist, is describing an encounter with refugees who are victims of torture. The story captures an extreme experience, but many staff, working with a variety of needs, will recognise the mixture of

101

feelings he describes. His description captures the disturbing tension that can be aroused in us all, including healthcare workers, as we face extreme need. The mixture of powerful feelings of compassion and responsibility, anxiety about how much patients need, the disturbing nature of their suffering and the urge to turn away can be overwhelming. This experience can be acute – in a particular encounter with an individual patient on a particular day – or chronic – evoked by working with profound needs, risks and vulnerabilities that do not go away over long periods of time, if at all. Work with the dependency and vulnerability of many people with intellectual disabilities, with the suffering and fragile lives of people with severe mental health difficulties, with the decline and decay that can characterise ageing, all confront staff with versions of these feelings.

On one level, the worker is pitched into these experiences by the nature of the needs of the patient. The experience can be amplified, however, by processes at work in the wider community. These processes influence not only the attitudes and feelings of the worker but also the resources offered to particular kinds of need, the policies that frame the work and the prospects for successful outcomes for patients – and staff. Staff working with patients from groups on the edge of kinship have not only to manage disturbing feelings aroused in themselves but also to encounter and work with others who are similarly affected.

Mixed feelings

The trouble with profound need is that it confronts us with the fear that we are not equipped to meet it – in terms of managing to face it, doing anything helpful about it, perhaps even surviving the encounter intact. There is an inevitable struggle with intense feelings, ranging from compassion through anxiety to overt anger and hostility. Such negative feelings can arise because we cannot bear the demand that need makes on us – so we end up hating the needy for it, and sometimes ourselves for feeling like that. The antipathy can extend to hating the other for the demands they make on material resources, blaming them for those demands, and finding ways to challenge their rights to make them. People in need can remind the rest of us of things we do not wish to acknowledge, about life, other people, ourselves – and we hate them for their reminders. Such hatred sits very uncomfortably alongside feelings of duty, compassion and concern.

The case of asylum seekers illustrates this vividly. The prospect of an uncontrolled invasion of people with the kind of needs described in Blackwell's vignette invokes fear and hostility – evidenced throughout the media and on the streets of many of our cities. An attempt to distinguish between undeserving ('bogus' in the public consciousness) and deserving ('genuine') asylum seekers is made. Society's feeling of rejection in the face of need then appears to influence both the process of assessing the claim of *all* asylum seekers and the treatment *both* 'genuine' and 'bogus' receive.

In her report *Fast and Fair?* the Parliamentary Ombudsman (2010, pp. 7–8) addressed the question of what kind of service should be provided by the UK Border Agency:

What should we expect from an effective system for the assessment of asylum applications? That applicants are told what to expect: that they are safe and properly supported while awaiting a decision, and that they receive a 'fast and fair' decision on their application. For those who are unsuccessful the expectation must be that, unless there is some other reason why they should be allowed to stay in the UK, they should promptly leave the country, or be removed as soon as is practicable.

In our experience the Agency are a very long way from achieving this.

Her investigation of complaints shows a system that was slow, unresponsive, intimidating and made errors about people's status. The very process of assessing eligibility appears to alienate, frighten and demean. Ashton & Moore (2009), clinicians working with asylum seekers, estimate that up to 30% of those turned down for asylum have, in fact, been tortured. It is unsurprising that traumatised people are less than comfortable 'qualifying themselves' for asylum by describing experiences of torture. Shame, and the effects of post-traumatic stress, are likely to inhibit such communication, even in the most humane of circumstances. If Ashton & Moore are right, the system does not appear to offer such humane circumstances, either in its processes or in the skills and sensitivity of its staff. The 'genuine' asylum seeker is being rejected along with people without grounds for asylum – and both categories are experiencing an inhumane system.

The Independent Asylum Commission confirms this view of the system, suggesting that is not yet fit for purpose, denies sanctuary to some who genuinely need it and ought to be entitled to it, is not firm enough in returning those whose claims are refused and is marred by inhumanity in its treatment of the vulnerable. The Commission sets these findings in a wider context:

we have an asylum system that purports to provide sanctuary, and yet the public have little understanding of what 'asylum' means, associate it – indelibly – with a range of negative and unrelated issues, and have little confidence in the asylum system itself. There is a profound disconnection in the public mind between the sanctuary they want the UK to provide and their perception of the asylum system. (Independent Asylum Commission, 2008, p. 6)

Unsuccessful applicants are particularly vulnerable. In a 2010 report, the Children's Commissioner, Sir Al Aynsley-Green, concluded that Yarl's Wood Immigration Removal Centre was 'no place for a child'. He said that the 1000 children detained in the centre each year often face 'extremely distressing' arrest and transportation procedures, and are subjected to prolonged and sometimes repeated periods of detention. Aynsley-Green also criticised failures to assess the mental well-being of children throughout the process, from arrival and during detention, even when children's behaviour had obviously changed in worrying ways. He raised 'significant concerns' about health services, and described one incident where a nurse failed to diagnose a broken arm in a young girl, who then waited 20 hours before being taken to hospital (Aynsley-Green, 2010). Despite commitments to end the practice of detaining children by both partners in the coalition government elected in May 2010, the practice continues as we write. There are also further examples of poor healthcare:

In any case, it appears that such centres are also 'no place for a human being': a pregnant woman detained at Yarl's Wood who was told by a midwife she could not find her baby's heartbeat was refused a scan for four days despite repeated requests and a high court order. She was already known to be suffering from depression after a miscarriage. (McVeigh, 2010)

Asylum seekers bring the traumas of loss and of mistreatment, the physical consequences of that mistreatment, and 'ordinary' healthcare problems (probably exacerbated by poverty, ill treatment and worse). Their ill-being is often extreme and complex; yet the deployment of the concepts of 'genuine' and 'bogus' and the consequent procedures seem to do nothing to help us contain rejecting feelings, manage hostility and offer the welcome and shelter we would want for ourselves in such circumstances. It appears that creating the category 'bogus' has neither helped British society manage its hostility towards 'the other' in great need, nor protected 'the genuine' from this hatred. A necessary procedure has become imbued with hostile and even brutal feelings that override compassion and justice.

In the case of asylum seekers, the defensive and brutal feelings are aroused by an encounter with 'outsiders'. There are situations where other groups, 'internal' to our community, arouse similar feelings. The brutal end of the spectrum is vividly expressed with dismaying frequency, particularly in the case of intellectual disabilities. In 2009, for example, Fiona Pilkington, mother of an 18-year-old daughter with intellectual disabilities, killed herself and her daughter after years of torment by local youths. In March 2010, a 64-year-old man with intellectual disabilities finally collapsed and died after 20 years of almost nightly taunting and harassment. Recent television documentaries, *Sticks and Stones* (Channel 4, 2010) and *Tormented Lives* (BBC1, 2010), have chronicled experiences of violence, harassment or neglectful indifference in the community. In the former, the carer of a person with intellectual disabilities said:

Care in the community was brought in so people are not locked away; they are cared for in the community and have normal lives. But they don't have normal lives. They are bullied and terrified, and the law is not protecting them.

Though brutality is by no means the only experience for people with intellectual disabilities or other vulnerable groups, the reality is that the mixture of responses they evoke includes such very unpalatable feelings, as well as generosity and concern. Citizens in general, and healthcare staff, resort to various mechanisms to deal with this discomfort – with the need to manage, to justify or to avoid the feelings involved. These 'strategies' may apparently be conscious, but they will almost always be accompanied and coloured by an unconscious element. They are dangerous when they are dominated by processes like the projection of dangerous, untrustworthy or malignant characteristics onto those in need. They are often conspicuously unsuccessful: they neither lead to effective response to need, nor mitigate the emotional ambiguity, let alone the hatred.

Inclusion and exclusion

In the face of such mixed feelings, society is torn between recognising the other as kin, and offering kindness and support, or rejecting their 'otherness', and punishing or ejecting them. Policies to promote the social inclusion of people from vulnerable groups tend to underestimate the degree to which this urge to hurt and eject is operating. The concept of stigma is often emptied of the sheer urge to obliterate that can be part of the response to vulnerable and needy difference. This urge can be expressed directly through violence, but is no less powerful when it is expressed in less obvious ways.

One mechanism at work is the process of *scapegoating*, where we project unwanted aspects of ourselves onto another person or group and then reject, hate or fear them (see Chapter 5, p. 77). This is an irrational, unconscious process, a process that allows us the illusion of ridding ourselves of things we are frightened to face – our vulnerability, our neediness, our violent feelings. The term *scapegoat* originates from the Old Testament. The story takes place on the Day of Atonement, when the prophet Aaron confessed all the sins of the children of Israel and ritually transferred them to a live goat, then sent the goat into the wilderness, bearing all these sins. The goat is literally excluded from the community, banished to the inhospitable environment of the wilderness. The community is, in turn, freed from its responsibilities and moral discomforts. Exclusion does not simply try to remove difficult people from among us but also seeks to banish unpalatable aspects of ourselves.

Society has traditionally responded to the challenging need and dependency of vulnerable groups by putting people into institutions. This included placing them in asylums and workhouses, but also involved imprisonment of very vulnerable people – as it does to this day. People with intellectual disabilities make up 2% of the UK population. Current estimates suggest that 7% of people in prison have an IQ of less than 70 and 20–30% of offenders have intellectual disabilities or learning difficulties that interfere with their ability to cope within the criminal justice system (Jacobson, 2008). Similarly, the best estimates suggest that 7% of sentenced male prisoners have a psychosis. The figure rises to 10% for males on remand and 14% for women, with many more having difficulties such as depression, anxiety and substance misuse (Appleby, 2010).

The problems with inclusion travel with people, and so transfer from the public world into institutions. Disturbing trends of neglect and abuse in asylums and similar residential settings have been reported for decades. It seems that the dynamics of institutional life conspire with the concentration of people with challenging needs to provoke neglectful and abusive behaviour, amplifying the tendency to rejection in society at large (Goffman, 1961). The joint report of the Healthcare Commission & Commission for Social Care Inspection (2006) into the care of people with intellectual disabilities in Cornwall, for example, found systemic neglect and abuse. Similar failures have been identified in other areas, such as Norfolk, and Sutton and Merton. Meanwhile, the toxic nature of psychiatric wards in many parts of the UK attracts ongoing concern, despite a number of policy initiatives that have addressed the issue (Mental Health Act Commission, 2009). In 2010, the President of the Royal College of Psychiatrists declared in his inaugural speech that many in-patient units were unsafe and uninhabitable, and that he would not be happy for himself or his relatives to be treated there (Bhugra, 2008).

Institutionalisation seems to express both benign concerns to protect and care, and impulses to 'eject' difficult people from the public sphere. The difficulty of including people with complex needs, the feelings aroused and the challenges involved in consistently meeting their needs humanely in society at large are transferred into these institutions. It is as if the institution itself becomes the scapegoat, bearing society's sins, absolving us of responsibility and making it easy to locate where any blame for our nastiness and limits lies. It (unsuccessfully, of course) carries the problems 'outside' society. It can become a place where, all too frequently, our darker responses, 'our sins', continue to find expression, conveniently hidden, and frequently amplified, behind closed doors.

There are many kinds of wilderness. Beyond the walls of the immigration centre, many unsuccessful applicants for asylum continue to live in the community. Because of the slowness and inefficiency of the state processes for appeal against the decision and removal, they enter a state of limbo that can last for years. Deprived of benefits and other rights, they are by law ineligible for secondary healthcare unless their condition is deemed an emergency, immediately life-threatening, or terminal.

The lesson is clear. The emotional challenge of inclusion, and the behaviours it evokes, do not go away, whether we establish systems to determine deservedness, as in the case of asylum seekers, or institutions to meet and contain difference, disturbance and need. Extremities of need inevitably evoke both compassionate and cruel feelings – in the same person, in groups, in institutions and in society. This reality becomes toxic if it is not managed – through acknowledgement and support for workers, as well as through policy and inspection systems. Without that acknowledgement and support, inspection will continue to find inhumanity, and the good intentions of policy will have limited effect.

Splitting

Being 'in two minds' about how to respond to otherness and need often expresses itself in *splitting*: the attempt to deny and remove the discomfort of having very mixed feelings through recourse to viewing the world as made up of objects deserving unambiguous love or hate (see Chapter 5, p. 77). A crucial truth about splitting is that, as a defence against anxiety about the nature and degree of need, it does not work. As we have seen, creating the legal category of the genuine asylum seeker does not take away the feelings of anxiety, hostility and fear, nor prevent them from being visited on all asylum seekers – 'genuine' and 'bogus'.

A similar splitting process can be seen in mental healthcare, where the complexity of mental distress can evoke sharp and oversimplifying distinctions, in society, in policy and in services. These splits and contradictions find their way into mental health practice and policy when the question of balancing the promotion of social inclusion, response to vulnerability, and the management of risk and dangerousness is considered. Despite, or perhaps because of, the fact that around 25% of the population will experience some form of mental health difficulty in their lifetime, mental ill health continues to arouse profound fears in the general population (MIND & Rethink, 2008).

In the face of challenging need and dependency, these fears are expressed both as fear of madness and as *fear of those who are mentally ill*. In that mental ill health is profoundly distressing, the first fear is rational, even if it often leads people to turn away from sufferers. It can, of course, enable empathy, and strengthen people's resolve to help. The second, which attributes dangerousness, is rarely justified, despite press and public hysteria about the relatively few cases where people with mental health difficulties harm others. Despite the substantial increase in homicides committed in the UK over the last 50 years of the 20th century, those attributable to people who were mentally ill remained stable, despite the closure of the asylums and a reduction in bed numbers (Taylor & Gunn, 1999). That truth does not seem to make much difference.

Staff must, of course, always work in a manner that includes an assessment of risk. In mental health, they must reconcile their caregiving responsibilities with their duty to intervene to restrict liberty. This tension is difficult in itself. However, when resources are tight, the problem is intensified. In the face of the potential split between concern for the person and protection of society, confronted by increasing need and the limits to their resources, staff are forced to ration their efforts, and they become increasingly anxious. The anxiety provokes practice skewed by 'risk aversion' (Pilgrim & Ramon, 2009). There is an inevitable pull towards risk assessments and coercive control, towards rationing and withholding resources from those who do not arouse anxiety, and away from open and welcoming kinship and compassionate practice. This is not just something that happens as a result of staff anxieties. Wider public anxiety infects inspection, management and governance, so that mental health workers are operating in a system that can be preoccupied with the view of people as dangerous. This pressure can be felt as very much at odds with being part of a service that promotes recovery and social inclusion. If policy makers and managers do not manage the tendency towards anxious splitting, then the work of staff drifts from imaginative compassion to a split between caution and control on the one hand, and underestimation of need and complexity on the other.

Such a drift is suggested by the facts that involuntary admissions to acute mental healthcare increased by 20% and the NHS use of private-sector medium-secure beds nearly trebled between 1996 and 2006 (Keown *et al*, 2008). At a time when the focus across healthcare – but especially in mental health – was care in the community, recourse to locking people away, in some of the most expensive settings around, mushroomed.

The problems of idealisation

Splitting always involves polarising between idealisation and denigration. Such splitting is frequently highly unstable – with individuals and society, through policy or preoccupation, swinging between contradictory positions. The community, staff or patients may be subject to these processes. Whenever they are at work, genuine attentiveness to people, as well as creative responses to their needs and aspirations, are undermined.

The laudable aim to reverse the trend towards institutionalisation expressed in current policies on intellectual disability (Department of Health, 2009*a*) can invoke serious underestimation of the difficulties in community life for service users, for those close to them and for the community. The woman quoted in the documentary earlier vividly expresses one aspect of this minimisation. It dangerously denies the cruelty and tendency to turn away in the community. But even without such extremes, life in the community is complicated and challenging for everyone, and it is easy to underestimate the difficulties involved, not just for people with intellectual disabilities, but also for frail older people and people with severe mental health difficulties.

Behind this underestimation can lie idealisation of the capabilities and potential of vulnerable people to cope in the community, as well as a parallel idealisation of that community. The first is often associated with a varyingly conscious tendency to blame people's disability on simplistic models of stigma and institutionalisation. The second leads to a minimisation of the sheer hard work involved, at times, in reading and responding to their needs and supporting them in leading fulfilling lives. As well as representing a doomed strategy for reducing anxiety and complexity, such idealisation is also useful in supporting unrealistic expectations of saving money. The outcome for patients can be exclusion, isolation or worse.

It is not difficult to see how such situations evolve. Specialist staff are understandably anxious about the challenges for their patients in the community. They can see themselves as the only ones capable of understanding and responding sensitively to the vulnerable individual. This can involve mistrust of, even contempt for, the capabilities of others, whether or not they are willing or able to respond kindly to people who have an intellectual disability or a mental illness. Realism about the limits of people and services is, of course, vital, but this dynamic can lead to a sort of default mistrust. This can undermine and restrict positive work with health and social care colleagues to improve practice and secure their patients' well-being. Where, for example, a carefully designed care plan to help a person with profound disabilities with their eating and drinking fails to be followed in a community setting, this can severely undermine the will of the specialist worker to collaborate. Vicious circles can then result.

Similarly, families, dedicated to a relative with a disability, and aware of a less than easy wider world, can fall into the same position, leading to mistrust of the community and professionals. The idealisation and denigration involved in both these cases can lead to overprotectiveness, diminished opportunities and reduced access to services and the world for the person in need.

These processes of splitting can be at work whether the group involved has intellectual difficulties, mental health problems or any other category of need that seriously challenges society's inclusiveness. The danger is that simplistic idealisation leads to people living materially, socially and emotionally impoverished and vulnerable lives, with poor health. Just as seriously, idealisation makes it hard, or impossible, for society or services to recognise or admit it. The complex task of engaging with real people, assessing their needs, evaluating risk, orchestrating resources, monitoring and responding, is undermined.

A dangerous effect of unmanaged splitting processes can be the failure of commissioners and providers of services to achieve an intelligent balance of care and support. In reality, health services and their partners need to ensure the right mix of priorities and resources, balancing the following:

- work to remove barriers to mainstream services
- the provision of an adequate range of specialist services
- risk minimisation and risk taking
- reliance on public support and protection from public neglect or abuse
- managing dependency and promoting independence.

When discussions and plans are influenced by urges to idealise or denigrate any element of this mix, or to minimise inconvenient truths, the danger is that the resulting service systems are ill equipped to respond to vulnerable people's needs. It is dangerous, for example, to base 'efficiency' plans for specialist healthcare services on idealistic assumptions that social care supports and opportunities for inclusion will be there, when resource limits and public sector cuts mean they will be scarce. Such unrealism is common. The resulting services are difficult environments in which to work. It is hard to maintain open attentiveness, empathy and responsive, responsible, kindness if services are affected by powerful splitting and polarising processes that encourage the denial of key aspects of the personhood and needs of people in vulnerable groups. The fact that these splits are played out at a policy level means staff also find themselves trying to reconcile the contradictions in organisational objectives, performance targets and scrutiny from seniors.

'Indirect discrimination'

The degree of denial and its consequences are illustrated vividly when the care of older people is considered. One of the benefits of the improvements in living conditions and healthcare in the UK has been the survival of more and more people into old age. The fastest population increase has been in the number of the 'oldest old'. In 1983, there were just over 600 000 people in the UK aged 85 and over. Twenty-five years later there were 1.3 million. By 2033 this group is projected to more than double again, to reach 3.2 million, or 5% of the total population. There is a gap, though, between life expectancy and how much of that is healthy, for large numbers of people.

Society is faced with the prospect of having to care for double the number of people with dementia (Department of Health, 2009b) and for increased demands for cancer care and treatment for long-term conditions such as diabetes, chronic obstructive pulmonary disease and heart disease. These trends have been known for years. Despite that knowledge, there has been a consistent failure to address the scale of need. Politicians, for example, have continued to fail to resolve the question of how personal care (vital for a life in the community) will be funded. Sometimes this failure has been accompanied by vivid signs of just how anxious and angry society is about this rising need. In the course of multi-party dialogue about this issue in February 2010, the Conservatives withdrew and began a poster campaign, caricaturing one option put on the table by Labour as a '£20,000 Death Tax'. This campaign neatly stirred up contempt and fear of taxation while playing on public fear of and wish to avoid the reality, and the costs, of ageing and dying.

Older people face discrimination across the health service. Carruthers & Ormondroyd (2009) suggested as much to the Secretary of State for Health in their report *Achieving Age Equality in Health and Social Care*. They drew heavily on work by the Centre for Policy in Ageing (2009a,b). They reported active and direct age discrimination – across a wide range of conditions and care delivery – in terms of access to or adequate funding for services needed by older people. They believed that much of this discrimination is based on ageist assumptions about the value of intervention into the illnesses of older people, about the comparative worth of the lives of younger and older people, and about how older people feel. Carruthers & Ormondroyd also described indirect discrimination – the disproportionate negative effect of policies, practices and management of care on older people.

Examining what this 'indirect discrimination' is sheds light on the predicament for older people themselves, but also has powerful messages relating to the circumstances of people with intellectual disabilities or mental health problems. The Centre for Policy in Ageing reports cite, by way of example, the way in which the pressure to discharge people from hospital can be at the expense of the right pace and detail of planning for life after the ward for older people. As people age, the capacity for *compensation*, the resilience and the ability to restore functioning in the face of illness, trauma or stress, decreases, in degree and in pace. This slowed, or impaired capacity for, recovery in older people makes them particularly vulnerable to the effects of drives for efficiency, for speeding up and systematising the journey through care. Although they may benefit from reduced waiting times, older people will lose out more than others through the reduction of staffing levels on wards, the pace at which staff are passing by, the fragmentation of care delivery in acute services, the speed of discharge processes, the shortness of primary care consultations. It takes *time* for the older patient and staff alike to establish the sense of attunement and trust described in Chapter 3. The inability to provide or sustain compassionate healthcare for older people was vividly illustrated in February 2011 by the Health Services Ombudsman, in her report into ten complaints (cases she felt were indicative of much wider failures). In a report full of distressing and shameful detail, she concluded that services had 'failed to provide even the most basic standards of care' (Health Services Ombudsman, 2011).

Experiences in in-patient care can be very bad, too, for people with intellectual disabilities and their carers. The Michael report (Michael, 2008) identified failures of acute healthcare for six people across the UK, whose deaths were highlighted in the Mencap report *Death by Indifference* (Mencap, 2007). Again, assumptions about the value and needs of the patients were seen to influence neglectful care. Recommendations for staff training, for systems and procedures have been turned into requirements from healthcare providers. But the underlying issue of whether sufficient time and staffing will be available to enable unrushed, attentive and sensitive dialogue with patients remains out of focus.

Time, and the attention and communication it allows, is increasingly unavailable in a modern NHS characterised by the drive to speed up treatment processes and to save money by providing the minimum numbers of staff. Time and human resource pressures frequently conspire to direct attention to procedures, to fragmented targets and tasks, and away from genuine engagement with patients. The specialisation of functions means that it is difficult to ensure continuity of relationships within which the person is understood. Often, neither the task nor the sympathetic relationship is even half-adequately addressed. In reality, older people, just like people with intellectual disabilities and other groups with complex needs, are experiencing indirect discrimination across the whole healthcare system, *because of its very culture of 'efficiency' and engineered processes.*

It is tempting to conclude that a fundamental denial is at work. It seems impossible to acknowledge that, even when fear, prejudice and hostility are managed, even when directives and models are proposed, these people and their complex needs *just do not seem to fit into our way of going about things.* This is frightening, to say the least, in light of the facts that 43% of the NHS budget was spent on people over 65 in 2003/4, and 65% of hospital beds were occupied by people in that age group, and that 25% of the population will experience mental health problems in their lifetime. Even if only a proportion find the system poorly geared to meet their needs, this is a lot of people not to fit in. The implications of requiring improved attention from primary, community and acute health services are consistently underestimated as a consequence of this denial. Inconveniently for both staff and patients, the needs of people in vulnerable groups on the edge of kinship require a lot of what the system has increasingly less of: unprejudiced attitudes, kindly concern, time and high levels of interpersonal skill. What is also wanted is a system that adjusts to their needs, rather than the other way round.

Promoting kinship at the edges

Members of groups on the edge of kinship, however much they inspire love, compassion, conscientiousness and concern, can be at the same time inconvenient and unwanted, even feared and hated. This reality is hard to face, and to address, especially as it is not going to go away, however much 'stigma' and 'discrimination' are challenged. As staff work with members of these groups, a core challenge is to remain open to them and their needs, to bear them in mind, despite anxiety and discomfort. Staff must then somehow manage to resist the temptation to split – to idealise or denigrate, to swing between trust and suspicion, to overestimate or underestimate patient or community resources. This temptation is personal, but it is also powerfully built into how society and health services respond to the patient's needs, and the pressures they put on the worker. At bottom, though, staff have constantly to deal with the lack of fit between the needs of their patients and the wider health and social care system. Often this will involve an encounter with frank discrimination, and almost always it will entail an engagement with culture and processes. The system frequently does not make available the resources patients need, and in fact too often goes about its business in ways that actually work against meeting their needs.

At a time of such pressure on public services, including the NHS, it is difficult to argue for more resources. Somehow, though, the time and space to build relationships with, and to develop and share understanding about, vulnerable people need to be found. Ways of strengthening the continuity of their care and supporting them as they encounter the many 'sharp edges' in wait for them in the community, and in the health and social care systems, are vital. Recognition of the dynamics at work at the edges of kinship may free up staff, may 'clear their heads', so that they can engage more compassionately with the real needs and aspirations of their patients. Managers can help, by resisting the urge to minimise the difficulties of the caring task, to idealise partial solutions, unreflectingly to demand contradictory priorities, to deny the shortcomings and limits that staff will encounter as they try to serve their patients.

References

Appleby, L. (2010) Offender health: the next frontier. *The Psychiatrist*, **34**, 409–410.

Ashton, L. & Moore, J. (2009) *Guide to Providing Mental Health Care Support to Asylum Seekers in Primary Care*. Royal College of General Practitioners.

Aynsley-Green, A. (2010) *Follow-Up Report to 'The Arrest and Detention of Children Subject to Immigration Control*. HMSO.

Bhugra, D. (2008) Quoted in 'Psychiatric patients feel lost and unsafe', by A. Hill, *Guardian*, 29 June 2008 (see http://www.guardian.co.uk/society/2008/jun/29/mentalhealth. health3, last accessed March 2011).

Blackwell, D. (2005) *Counselling and Psychotherapy with Refugees*. Jessica Kingsley.

Carruthers, I. & Ormondroyd, J. (2009) *Achieving Age Equality in Health and Social Care*. HMSO.

Centre for Policy in Ageing (2009a) *Ageism and Age Discrimination in Secondary Health Care in the United Kingdom*. HMSO.

Centre for Policy in Ageing (2009b) *Ageism and Age Discrimination in Primary and Community Health Care in the United Kingdom*. HMSO.

Department of Health (2009a) *Valuing People Now*. HMSO.

Department of Health (2009b) *Dementia Strategy*. HMSO.

Goffman, E. (1961) *Asylums: Essays on the Condition of the Social Situation of Mental Patients and Other Inmates*. Penguin.

Healthcare Commission & Commission for Social Care Inspection (2006) *Joint Investigation into the Care of People with Learning Disabilities at Cornwall Partnership NHS Trust*. HMSO.

Health Services Ombudsman (2011) *Care and Compassion? A Report of the Health Services Ombudsman on Ten Investigations into NHS Care for Older People*. HMSO.

Independent Asylum Commission (2008) *Saving Sanctuary: The First Report of Conclusions and Recommendations*. IAC.

Jacobson, J. (2008) *No-One Knows*. Prison Reform Trust.

Keown, P., Mercer, G. & Scott, J.(2008) Retrospective analysis of hospital episode statistics, involuntary admissions under the MHA 1983, and number of psychiatric beds in England 1996–2006. *BMJ*, **337**, a1837.

McVeigh, K. (2010) Pregnant women at Yarl's Wood denied hospital scandals despite baby scare. *Guardian*, 8 October.

Mencap (2007) *Death by Indifference*. Mencap.

Mental Health Act Commission (2009) *The Mental Health Act Commission Annual Report*. HMSO.

Michael, J. (2008) *Healthcare for All*. HMSO.

MIND & Rethink (2008) *Time to Change Campaign*. See http://www.time-to-change.org. uk (last accessed March 2011).

Parliamentary Ombudsman (2010) *Fast and Fair? Report by the Parliamentary Ombudsman on the UK Border Agency*. TSO (The Stationery Office).

Pilgrim, D. & Ramon, S. (2009) English mental health policy under New Labour. *Policy and Politics*, **37**, 273–288.

Taylor, P. & Gunn, J. (1999) Homicides by people with mental illness: myth and reality. *British Journal of Psychiatry*, **174**, 9–14.

CHAPTER 8

The end of life

The best we can hope for is harmonious decline. (Raymond Tallis, 2005, p. 275)

Healthcare has two main objectives: to prolong life and to alleviate suffering. There are times when these are in conflict and important judgements have to be made. Kindness involves facing up to the reality of such tensions and responding with wisdom and sensitivity. Unkindness is often linked to the failure of staff to manage this well and the failure of the system to support them in this.

We find it hard to let people die. Death is a modern taboo, a dreaded unknown that strikes or creeps up on us and finds us unrehearsed. This contrasts with the past, when dying was a relatively common public event. Before the First World War, the average 16-year-old would have seen six people die. Now it is common to be 50 and never to have seen a corpse (Smith, 2010). Most of us find ways to evade the shocking but incontrovertible truth that human life will forever remain a condition with a 100% mortality rate. And modern culture colludes with this denial, creating a sort of collective manic defence against both the inevitability and uncertainty of death.

The *Economist* has argued that the uncontrollable costs of US healthcare are driven by fear of death (cited by Smith, 2010). Anton Obholzer, a medical psychoanalyst and consultant to organisations, suggested that the health service should more accurately be called a 'keep-death-at-bay' service:

In the unconscious, there is no such concept as 'health'. There is, however, a concept of 'death' and in our constant attempt to keep this anxiety repressed, we use various unconscious defensive mechanisms, including the creation of social systems to serve the defensive function. (Obholzer, 1994, p. 171)

What does this mean for patients, carers and staff? The majority of people who die in the UK do so in acute hospitals, usually following a chronic illness, and are over the age of 75 years. Most people would prefer to die in their own home, even though less than 20% do, with a similar proportion dying in care homes and very few dying in hospices (Department of Health, 2008).

Death in hospital

Dealing with death in a hospital aiming at keeping people alive is complicated. Alex Paton wrote in the *BMJ* about his wife's death and the difficulty the 'system' had in 'letting her go'. Despite the fact that at 85 she had multiple disabilities, despite providing the staff with an 'advance directive' stating her wish to the contrary, she was resuscitated after a cardiac arrest. The family eventually decided to take her home but were required to sign her out against medical advice. Even at home, while she was peacefully passing the last few days of her life surrounded by family, there was pressure to embark on another series of blood tests, 'just to make sure there is nothing treatable' (Paton, 2009).

Recent reports from NCEPOD found that aggressive but unavailing cancer treatment was still being given to some patients too near to the end of their life (NCEPOD, 2008) and that hospital care did not always switch in a sensitive and timely fashion from sustaining life to allowing natural death (NCEPOD, 2009). The latter study included over 3000 patients who died within 96 hours of admission. Even in the subgroup of those who were not expected to survive the admission, in 16.9% there was no evidence of any discussion of treatment limitation between the healthcare team and either the patients or relatives. The report highlights examples where healthcare professionals were judged not to have the skills required to care for patients nearing the end of their lives. This was particularly so in relation to a lack of the ability to identify patients approaching the end of life, inadequate implementation of end-of-life care, and poor communication with patients, relatives and other healthcare professionals.

From a physician's view, Raymond Tallis describes how the fear of reprisal can lead to patients being subjected to endless tests and attention by specialists, just so they and their families believe that 'everything has been done' – a practice he describes as 'clinically and morally lazy' (Tallis, 2005, p. 106). There is some evidence from the USA (cited by Tallis) that doctors were making decisions in favour of resuscitation because of fear of litigation, in full knowledge that such efforts would be futile.

Doctors are reluctant even to talk about dying, to move the dialogue with the patient or the family into another gear, for fear of being told that they are 'writing the patient off'. (Tallis, 2005, pp. 106–107)

Most patients and their loved ones are unaware of what the process of cardiopulmonary resuscitation (CPR) entails. The situation is graphically described by another physician, John Saunders:

At its best, CPR is the gift of life: chest compression, ventilation, intravenous medication and defibrillation followed by years of productive and fulfilled being. At its worst, it offers a scenario of vomit, blood and urine, then a confused, brain-damaged twilight, breathlessness from a failing ventricle, pain from rib fractures, until expiring in thrall to the full panoply of intensive care or forgotten in the long darkness of the persistent vegetative state. No humane doctor would consider this a good death, nor would any poet, priest, painter, musician or novelist use images of CPR to represent the Good Death. Rather, the images are more likely to be those of the factory: death in the industrial age. (Saunders, 2001)

This bleak scenario has been assertively, but inconclusively, addressed over the past decade. Since 2001, for example, all NHS trusts have been required to have a resuscitation policy which includes DNAR (do not attempt resuscitation) orders; yet according to the 2009 NCEPOD report, only 30% of the subgroup of terminal patients not expected to survive admission had such an order. Likewise, the Department of Health's *End of Life Care Strategy* (2008) pushes for coordinated development of palliative care teams, both in the community and in the acute sector; but NCEPOD (2009) found that 81% of patients who died within 96 hours of hospital admission had no such involvement. Even in the subgroup specifically allocated terminal care, only 50% had involvement of a palliative care team. So there is a long way to go.

Understanding the problem

Modern affluent society is particularly uncomfortable with the reality of death, a discomfort that makes it a difficult area for both healthcare staff and patients and their families. Some doctors and nurses feel anxious about engaging in a conversation about death and prefer to avoid it. They adopt a more comfortable, task-centred approach, focusing on the disease process and the technicalities of intervention rather than risk emotional, inter-personal contact. At the same time, some patients and their families find it difficult to face the thought of imminent death and understandably want 'everything possible' to be done, reinforcing the pressure on staff to adopt aggressive treatment approaches, however minimal the possibility of 'cure'.

Concern to avoid ageism can also lead to unnecessary intervention. While there can be a narrow line between informed empathy and overprotective or negative prejudice, it is important to be able to distinguish between 'ageism' and 'age-differentiated attitudes'. The latter are based on the 'thoughtful recognition of age differences' and an understanding of the ageing process (Carruthers & Ormondroyd, 2009).

Media coverage of isolated incidents of malpractice means that mistrust of professionals is more prevalent than it used to be, creating fertile ground for suspicion and defensiveness on all sides. Successful litigation is still rare in the UK but looms large in professional minds; and being under scrutiny in an official inquiry is a long and frightening process. It is easier to bypass the 'difficult conversation', to avoid getting into conflict and to see oneself as a cog in the wheel of the keep-death-at-bay system. The trouble is, where everyone is geared to prolonging life, every death represents failure and attempts to keep these feelings at a distance lead to more defensiveness and feed into the vicious circle.

Keeping life and death in mind

Psychoanalysts talk about *part-object relating* to describe the situation where relating to another as a whole person (*whole-object relating*) causes such high anxiety that, unconsciously, we defend ourselves and relate to only one aspect. Medical achievement and progress are reliant on the capacity to distance oneself from pain, mess and fear in order to think objectively, but to do this with awareness. Related to this is the ability to cut off from the whole picture and focus on a specific part – most obviously, surgeons must be able to narrow their focus to the organs in front of them during an intricate operation.

Nevertheless, success is also dependent on the capacity to be *bifocal*, to switch flexibly between the narrow gaze and the whole panoramic picture. Trends in healthcare make this hard. With increasing medical specialism and narrower realms of expertise, there is huge pressure to focus on part objects at the expense of the whole person, sometimes, even, to the point of missing the primary diagnosis. Someone needs to be holding a more complete picture of the person in mind, and drawing this to the attention of all involved. This includes the *prognosis*, which may be that the person is dying, and needs help to go through that experience. In the past, GPs would play a key role in providing continuity, overviewing and coordinating a patient's care. These days, the connection between GP and patient, in terms of the time spent together and the continuity of attention through complex journeys in the healthcare system, has become harder to maintain and urgently needs protecting and strengthening. Patients want to be seen as the persons they are, beyond symptoms that require intervention, and this perspective needs to include their mortality. There is a strong argument for providing specialist care coordination to help bring this kind of recognition into the work of those treating the dying.

We have seen in earlier chapters that fragmentation in the system can be amplified by the high levels of anxiety experienced and the unconscious psychological mechanisms that people erect to defend themselves. Nowhere is this more pertinent than in care at the end of life, which can so easily arouse feelings in everyone of personal loss and fear of mortality. The NCEPOD (2009, p. 79) study described, for example, a number of cases of terminal patients admitted to hospital inappropriately in response to acute symptoms, without due consideration of the patients' overall condition or indeed their wishes. Of course, this could be partly about available resources but, on a psychological level, the GPs may have found it easier to focus on the symptoms in isolation than think about the symptoms in relation to the overall situation of the patients and the fact that they were nearing death.

Another medical intervention that can create dilemmas and provoke differences of opinion between patients, relatives and professionals is the use of artificial feeding systems in the care of the dying. The Royal College of Physicians & British Society of Gastroenterology (2010) have criticised the overuse of such systems. They found evidence of poor practice and suggested that patients are too often put on such systems in hospitals for the convenience of staff or because of an overly defensive response to the reality of the patients' condition.

Facing up to death

There are, of course, areas of good practice, particularly in hospices, where palliative care is the explicit objective. In facing the fact that they are working with people who are dying, all involved are freed up to make the last stages of life meaningful and to minimise the suffering involved. In palliative-care settings, staff and patients are clear about this reality, and the scene is set for creative, collaborative relationships with a shared focus. Staff who work in such settings, rather like those who work with asylum seekers, tend to share similar values and have a shared sense of purpose, the bedrock being the partnership sought between healthcare staff and the patient. But a strong ideology can bring its own problems. Peter Speck, a hospital chaplain, warns against the common expectation that good care will make for a 'good death': 'death is not just sad or beautiful; it can be ugly, painful and frightening' (Speck, 1994, p. 94). He then cautions against the danger of 'chronic niceness', the desire to be the perfect carer and do everything possible to ensure that the person nearing death has 'quality time':

While there is little doubt that hospice staff are caring and dedicated people, one of the dangers which face them, and others who work long term with dying people, is that of 'chronic niceness', whereby the individual and the organisation collude to split off and deny the negative aspects of caring daily for the dying. There is a collective fantasy that the staff are nice people, who are caring for nice dying people, who are going to have a nice death in a nice place. This protects everyone from facing the fact that the relationship between the carers and the dying can often arouse very primitive and powerful feelings which are disturbingly not-nice. (Speck, 1994, p. 97)

In these situations, the danger is that not-so-nice feelings get split off and displaced on to patients' relatives, colleagues or managers – all of which can have a detrimental effect on patient care. Another scenario, more common in settings where there is less shared philosophy and palliative care is not the explicit objective, is a potentially unhelpful split between medical and nursing staff, with doctors typically holding the disease-focused, life-saving approach and nurses focusing on the relief of suffering. This can be fine if the division of labour is complementary and the different groups are working in partnership. Too often, though, the anxiety in the system amplifies such tendencies and a chronic destructive rivalry creeps in, which again can have a detrimental effect on patient care.

In settings like hospices, where the philosophy is explicit, it is much easier to work with the inherent anxieties, and understand and contain situations where anxiety is displaced and projected. Sensitively managing the end of a patient's life in a more general setting, particularly when staff are dealing with a mixed group of emergencies, is problematic in many ways. As we have seen, it is hard for staff racing from one patient to another not to become exclusively focused on saving lives. Alleviating suffering can then feel like a low priority. Discussing the matter of death and dying with the patient and family is sometimes avoided completely, often with the rationalisation that the patient does not really want to know. More often, a discussion about death takes place but the personal nature of the conversation is minimised by the overuse of technical information and statistics; or the bare facts are spoken bluntly by the staff member, who then leaves quickly to avoid the painful impact of the news.

Medical and nursing school curricula have included palliative care for many years, not to mention communication skills, including role-plays of breaking bad news. Nevertheless, a disturbing number of doctors and nurses in the NCEPOD (2009) study (29% and 18% respectively) reported having received no undergraduate training in palliative care. Even if it was properly covered, it is difficult to anticipate fully the real-life situation, in an environment where everyone's anxiety is high. It seems likely that while younger generations of healthcare staff may be more skilled than their predecessors in talking through difficult issues with patients, the anxiety around death in society generally and in hospitals specifically has increased, for the reasons mentioned earlier, making it more difficult to discuss.

Kindness at the end of life

The Department of Health's helpful *End of Life Care Strategy* (2008) identifies as key areas of action raising the profile of end-of-life care and changing attitudes to death and dying in society, as well as education and training of generalist healthcare staff. A number of the other themes identified resonate with our theme of kindness and kinship. There is encouragement to identify people approaching the end of life, to allow a discussion about the person's preferences for the place and type of care needed; to assess the needs and wishes of the person and to agree the subsequent care plan with the person and carers. There is encouragement to increase provision of services in the community, hopefully preventing emergency admissions to hospitals and enabling more people approaching the end of their lives to live and die in the place of their choice – often at home with their family. There is recognition of the need to empower generalist clinicians to manage pain and other symptoms in the last hours of life and to coordinate care after death. There is the commitment to involve and support carers in the provision of care.

Various care pathways, such as the Liverpool Care Pathway (see http://www.liv.ac.uk/mcpcil/liverpool-care-pathway), have been developed to help improve end-of-life care. While it is hoped that these will succeed by providing a common framework and developing inexperienced staff, the NCEPOD report (2009) warns against 'the act of dying becoming over medicalised and process driven' and argues that 'good quality end of life care can equally well be provided by committed and compassionate individuals who are experienced in the care of the dying'. The National Audit Office's (2008) report *End of Life Care* found that positive experiences of care were often linked to being treated by staff who understood, appreciated and empathised with the end-of-life situation. Increasingly, there is agreement that the patient's wishes should be respected and that everyone deserves dignity and respect during their final days. Advance care plans or directives seek to make clear a person's wishes in anticipation of a gradual deterioration in their condition, which may result in a loss of capacity to make decisions or to communicate their wishes to others. Putting these principles into action will require supporting staff to manage and process their personal feelings, and to reconcile patient death to a healthcare system anxiously working to preserve life.

Another thought on intelligent kindness and how it might inform end-of-life care is again related to the idea of kinship. It is the obvious observation that patients in hospital are not on their own, but part of a group of patients. Anyone who is conscious and in hospital for more than a few hours is well aware of this. Even very ill patients often have an awareness of the other patients in nearby beds, sometimes very acute even when they cannot speak, and in some cases lasting friendships are made. Feelings from sympathy to frank irritation arise and those left behind may well be affected and depressed by a death. Staff often answer questions about other patients with evasive platitudes, partly rationalised by a duty of confidentiality, but in some settings there is more awareness that relationships formed at such times can be deeply meaningful and that their loss needs to be acknowledged and marked in some way.

Intelligent kindness surely demands that healthcare staff are authentic and help patients towards the truth, even if very gently in some instances. By encouraging people to face the inevitable reality of death and think through and discuss various end-of-life scenarios, the unhelpful taboo on death may begin to lessen. How can thinking about kinship and kindness help with this struggle?

The critical challenge is explicitly to recognise that dying has become something the general social 'family' – especially in affluent societies – 'just doesn't talk about', despite its universality. As a result, there is an absence of language, of 'etiquette' and of forums within which to discuss dying. Closely related to facing this 'family secret' is to acknowledge the lengths society goes to place the responsibility for life and death (especially life!) at the door of clinical staff – to recruit them to keeping death at bay. With such acknowledgement, room begins to be made for citizens generally, and healthcare staff in particular, to be able to think about and address the reality of death. A guiding principle that may prevent denial or omnipotent intervention is that we are all kin when it comes to death. Helping staff to put themselves in the place of the dying, and think about what they would want in the range of circumstances the dying face, will tend to mitigate the effects of denial, feelings of omnipotence and inappropriate responses. When this act of imagination then colours the questions and reflections that take place in the conversation between healthcare workers and between them and the patient or patient's family, it can bypass accusations of 'doctors playing God' or relatives feeling guilty that they are agreeing to a death sentence. It opens up the possibility of a collaborative, empathic process leading to a gentler consensus.

References

Carruthers, I. & Ormondroyd, J. (2009) *Achieving Age Equality in Health and Social Care.* HMSO.

Department of Health (2008) *End of Life Care Strategy.* HMSO.

National Audit Office (2008) *End of Life Care.* London: HMSO.

NCEPOD (2008) *Systemic Anti-Cancer Therapy: For Better, For Worse?* National Enquiry into Patient Outcomes and Deaths. Available at http://www.ncepod.org.uk/2008sact.htm (last accessed March 2011).

NCEPOD (2009) *Deaths in Acute Hospitals: Caring to the End?* National Confidential Enquiry into Patient Outcomes and Death. Available at http://www.ncepod.org.uk/2009dah.htm (last accessed March 2011).

Obholzer, A. (1994) Managing social anxieties in public sector organisations. In *The Unconscious at Work* (eds A.Obholzer & V. Zagier Roberts), pp.169–178. Brunner–Routledge.

Paton, A. (2009) Letting go. (Personal view.) *BMJ*, **339**, b4982.

Royal College of Physicians & British Society of Gastroenterology (2010) *Oral Feeding Difficulties and Dilemma: A Guide to Practical Care, Particularly Towards the End of Life.* RCP.

Saunders, J. (2001) Perspectives on CPR: resuscitation or resurrection? *Clinical Medicine*, 1, 457–460.

Smith, R. (2010) Death becomes us. Review of two books on death. *BMJ*, **340**, c79.

Speck, P. (1994) Working with dying people. In *The Unconscious at Work* (eds A.Obholzer & V. Zagier Roberts), pp. 94–100. Brunner–Routledge.

Tallis, R. (2005) *Hippocratic Oaths: Medicine and Its Discontents.* Atlantic Books.

Part III
The organisation of kindness

CHAPTER 9

Unsettling times

The NHS workforce is now accustomed to being told every couple of years that they are about to face the biggest overhaul since the beginning of the health service and that the process of modernisation is only entering its stride, and that they are about to face 'unsettling times'. (Tony Blair, in 2000)

Maintaining the virtuous circle of kinship and kindness outlined in Chapter 3 involves understanding and managing individual, team and systems dynamics and relationships. But it must also address the influence of *culture* on the attitudes, emotions and practice of staff. Everybody in an organisation is working within what Larry Hirschhorn, former President of the International Society for the Psychoanalytic Study of Organizations, called 'the workplace within' (Hirschhorn, 1988) and David Armstrong, a principal consultant at the Tavistock Consultancy Service, London, calls 'the organisation in the mind' (Armstrong, 2005). This is the idea that everyone builds up a kind of internal working model of the organisation, part conscious, part unconscious, which profoundly colours their experience, how they understand their tasks, manage themselves in their roles and work with others. The way in which the tasks, priorities, anxieties and relationships are viewed and managed makes up the culture of an organisation and this is, in turn, *internalised* by everyone concerned.

A positive therapeutic culture will reinforce our virtuous circle. Building such a culture requires hard work over time, with continuous attention to a wide range of pressures, management of difficult feelings, and the development of agreements, norms and understandings between staff. This work, though, is strongly influenced by powerful cultural factors arising from the way the NHS is understood and organised as a whole and by how this is translated into the culture of the organisations in which people work. Unmanaged and unmitigated, these factors add impetus to the vicious circle that pulls healthcare away from effective kindness, and undermines therapeutic culture.

Several trends have powerful effects on the culture of care:
- the approach to system and structural change
- the market philosophy in healthcare

- the industrialisation of healthcare
- the regulation of performance of healthcare.

Before examining how these factors influence the culture of kindness, it is helpful to understand what is involved in preserving kinship and mutuality in human groups, and just how vulnerable such cultures can be.

A lesson from ethology

Informative work with non-human primates led by Michael Chance (1988) illuminates this issue powerfully. Like many researchers, Chance was concerned to discover what we share with these zoological relatives and what distinguishes us from them – 'what drags us back and what potentially sets us free by setting free our intelligence?' (Chance, 1988, p. 1). He described three distinct mental modes of social functioning, the agonic, the hedonic and the agonistic, based on comparing and categorising the structures of similar societies of non-human primates.

In the *agonic mode*, characteristic of hierarchical societies, such as African savannah baboons, individuals are primarily concerned with self-security, with warding off potential threats and with maintaining their status in the hierarchy. Members of the group become either authoritarian or subservient. They are preoccupied with *inhibiting* overt expressions of aggressive conflict, which means tension and arousal remain at a characteristically high level. The result is a social culture that inhibits individual development and restricts intelligence.

In the *hedonic mode*, individuals are freer to form a network of personal relationships that offer mutual support, enabling attention to be released from self-protective needs, thereby giving free rein to intelligence and creativity and a virtuous circle of reciprocity. In the hedonic societies typical of the wild chimpanzee and gorilla, much time is spent nurturing social relations. This includes competitive play, which is often followed by displays of tenderness, gentle touching and kissing. Such behaviour is both reassuring and rewarding because it reduces tension and arousal. Apart from short-lived bursts of excitement, levels of tension and arousal in the hedonic mode are characteristically low. Hedonic social interaction promotes self-confidence, empathic cooperation and reality-based intelligence. The hedonic mode seems to capture the virtuous circle of kind and attentive behaviours outlined in Chapter 3, but, as we will see, is very vulnerable under pressure.

The third form of relating described by Chance is the *agonistic mode*, where individuals simply fight it out among themselves. The violence often becomes ritualised, but still threatens to consume all-important group resources and is thus disadvantageous in terms of overall group survival.

Extrapolating from groups of primates, Chance hypothesised that human groups may become stuck in the agonic or hedonic mode, or unconsciously move back and forth between them. Each mode predisposes individuals and groups to deploy their attention in distinct ways, so that they are either prevented from or enabled to develop their intelligence.

Of particular interest are studies that have observed hedonic societies of primates that have changed dramatically to become agonic or even agonistic (overtly destructive). The best-known example is the breakdown in social order among chimpanzees at the Gombe Stream Reserve in Tanzania. Researchers, eager to engage these primates, provoked disarray in their peer relations by using bananas as an enticement and a reward (Goodall, 1965). This practice created intense competition and, after it had been in existence for some time, one group started hounding and killing members of another group. The hedonic relations that had previously existed broke down. One theory about this is that prolonged and frustrated competition reduced the opportunities for the mutual reassuring and affiliative gestures typical of wild chimpanzees. This then led to arousal being sustained at a raised level. At the same time, it altered the type of attention that characterised their relationships from essentially one of *awareness of* rather than *reaction to* each other (Power, 1988). When the opportunity to practise mutually reassuring rituals was prevented through a critical period of prolonged competitive provocation, the network of social attention underlying the social relations collapsed. Hedonic groups are particularly vulnerable to destructive influences. This is because, unlike agonic societies, they do not have the rigid in-built structure that will reassert itself after the social links are temporarily broken. The individuals in a hedonic group have not learnt to inhibit the violent and aggressive impulses that keep the highly tense and aroused agonic individual in check. The infrastructure of mutually dependent hedonic social relations is constantly maintained by reassurance and tender appeasement, reinforced by arousal reduction. This enables the relations between one generation and the next to be smoothly integrated. In Gombe, this integration was broken by continuous competitive provocation, leaving the chimpanzees wide open to social destruction. An important lesson is that hedonic relations, though they liberate creative intelligence, are extremely vulnerable, particularly in the context of an overcrowded world with limited resources. A kind and attentive society of primates is dependent on an ongoing reward cycle of active reciprocal kindnesses.

Chance's ideas offer a frame for further understanding of the alarming findings of the social experiments summarised in Chapter 5. These experiments spoke eloquently of how authority, conformism, threat and risk can drive behaviour towards brutality and how anxiety and limited resources can provoke splitting and unproductive disputes between people and teams. The lessons from non-human primates point powerfully to the vulnerability of the culture of kindness and to some of the dynamics that can fatally undermine it. At the heart of the issue is how (hedonic) attentiveness to and nurture of the other can be so easily subverted, even replaced, by uncontrolled (agonic) self-protective or status-driven attitudes or, worse, by (agonistic) brutality.

It appears the culture of healthcare is similarly vulnerable. In the inquiry report into the alarming mortality rates and appaling clinical conditions at Mid-Staffordshire NHS Trust, the new medical director was *praised* for saying 'Our job is to treat patients. That is all there is to it' (Francis, 2010, p. 402). How have we come to reach such a state of affairs that this simple statement sounds so radical?

'Re-disorganisation'

In Part II, we began to explore the pressures on individuals and teams in the modern health service and the importance of them being helped to focus on their role in order to manage conflicting pressures. Probably the most frequent topic of discontent among staff in the NHS is the culture of constant change, often referred to scathingly by staff as 're-disorganisation' (Smith *et al*, 2001). The scale of the change culture is summed up in an editorial in the *BMJ*:

Over the past 30 years, governments have reached repeatedly for structural reorganizations of both the NHS and the Department of Health. They have created, merged and abolished health bodies and distributed service, functional and geographical responsibilities in different ways. Reorganisation has often been cyclical, with new governments or ministers reinventing structural arrangements that their predecessors abolished, seemingly unaware of or uninterested in past reorganizations. Reorganization has happened frequently – with at least 15 identifiable major structural changes in three decades, or one every two years or so. And reorganization has been rapid, with changes often being initiated in advance of formal legislative approval, the details of reforms being worked out as they are implemented, and the timetable for hasty consultation being a matter of weeks or months. (Walshe, 2010)

In addition to the major reorganisations, there have been changes in commissioning arrangements, merging and demerging of trusts, breaking and forming new partnerships, and the restructurings that automatically seem to follow the frequent changes of chief executive. Staff have also been close to overwhelmed by the mushrooming of official top-down policies, guidelines and audits and major strategic changes in direction in relation to the clinical management of certain patient groups. Furthermore, they have faced huge changes to professional career planning and ways of working, changes that have not always been well managed or led.

Stability and consistency have been further undermined by multiple changes at service level, including 're-engineering' of teams, changes to contracts, bed reductions and the shifting of resources from secondary to primary care. It is *not* that all such change should not be made. But no other successful business or industry has been in such a state of permanent disequilibrium and (almost without exception) unfinished processes of change for so long. How can any stable compassionate, task and patient-focused culture survive in the face of such disturbances? The lessons from primates indicate that calm and stability are required to nurture and sustain kindness and creativity. If that appears a recipe for stagnation and complacency, then at least the way change is managed requires rethinking.

Top-down change

Change tends to get rushed through, with poor planning and little thought about its likely effect on existing systems. Having reassured the British public throughout the election campaign and agreed in the coalition programme for government to 'stop the top-down reorganizations of the NHS that have got in the way of patient care' (HM Government, 2010) the white paper, *Equity and Excellence: Liberating the NHS* (Department of Health, 2010) was produced, at speed, only 7 weeks after the formation of the coalition government in May 2010. It, and the Health and Social Services Bill it foreshadowed, introduced the most radical changes in the organisation of the NHS for decades – perhaps since its foundation – including the abolition of previous commissioning arrangements through PCTs and the transfer of these responsibilities to consortia of GPs and much more competition among service providers. Leaving aside the lack of democratic mandate for its proposals and major misgivings expressed by professional groups and academic experts in health policy and management, there is general agreement that the intention is for far-reaching and profound change that will undoubtedly cause massive upheaval. In this respect, the stort 'pause' in the process announced in April 2011 is welcome. It remains to be seen whether changes to the pace or direction emerge.

In a *BMJ* editorial, it was estimated that every major NHS restructuring puts the NHS back 3 years. They do not achieve the stated objectives of increasing efficiency, reducing management costs and channelling a greater proportion of resources to the front line (Walshe, 2010). Transition costs are always underestimated and intended savings rarely realised (National Audit Office, 2010), while management costs have grown steadily in the NHS over the past 30 years, regardless of reorganisations.

Why do politicians and those in power beneath them feel a need to overwhelm the system with changes of direction and structure rather than putting their energy and the country's resources into improving the systems already in place? This is not even about the government changing hands. The Labour government in 2000, for example, set out a road map for the next 10 years in *The NHS Plan*, with a strengthened approach to targets and performance management (Department of Health, 2000). Some 12 months later, before the approach had had a chance to deliver improvements, the emphasis changed to promoting choice and competition (Ham, 2009). There is evidence that large-scale change programmes are never linear and are often characterised by the so-called 'J curve', in which there is a dip in performance before improvements occur. Constant revolution, then, also means constant failure. Politicians, however, seem unable to learn from history and are

129

condemned to repeat the mistakes of the past, quite unable to allow time for the changes to become embedded – let alone properly evaluated – before upheaving the system again. The irrationality of this pattern suggests that reality cannot be fully faced and psychological defence mechanisms are in operation.

Social defences

In previous chapters, we saw how individuals and teams have a tendency to organise in ways that minimise the conscious experience of anxiety. The behaviour of large organisations can be explored from a similar perspective. A famous study of nurses in the 1950s (Menzies Lyth, 1959) sought to understand why nurses resigned from their profession in such high numbers. It showed that the stresses of nursing, and the intimate relationship it demanded with patients, made an impact on the organisation of care, leaving those closest to patients exposed to emotional pressures that most senior staff and managers were defended against. Menzies Lyth felt that the work of nursing – what she called the *objective situation* – because it involves physical and emotional contact with illness, pain, suffering and death, arouses feelings and thoughts associated with the 'deepest and most primitive levels of the mind' (1988, p. 47).

She proceeded to show how the organisation of the hospital can be seen as being consciously and unconsciously structured round the evasion of this anxiety. The observations which drew her to these conclusions included a range of interacting phenomena. She identified the process of splitting up the nurse–patient relationship by breaking the workload down into a list of tasks and dividing each nurse's time between 30 patients. She observed depersonalisation and categorisation (e.g. referring to the patients as 'the liver in bed 10' rather than by name) and the detachment and denial of feelings. She noted the attempt to eliminate decisions by ritual task performance and to reduce the weight of responsibility in decision-making by checks and counter-checks. She found purposeful obscurity in the formal redistribution of responsibility, both idealisation and underestimation of personal development possibilities, and avoidance of change. Importantly, she saw that the social defence system

prevents the individual from realising to the full her capacity for concern, compassion and sympathy, and for action based on these feelings that would strengthen her belief in the good aspects of herself and her capacity to use them. (Menzies Lyth, 1959; 1988, p. 75)

Menzies Lyth proposed that the success and viability of a social institution are intimately connected with the techniques it uses to contain anxiety. In the intervening years, these ideas have been developed, with account being taken of the *goodness of fit* between organisational structures on the one hand and the emotional demands of healthcare work on the other.

Unconscious drivers of change?

The idea that the organisation of a hospital is defensive, with the unconscious purpose of stopping those who work in it – particularly those in charge – from feeling the emotional pain and anxiety associated with the work, is an important one. There is certainly evidence that major structural change keeps senior managers and board members detached from the front line of healthcare (Healthcare Commission, 2007; Francis, 2010). Could it be that the constant restructuring of the health service fulfils a similar function to those nursing rituals observed in the Menzies Lyth study? That the unremitting process is in part a *social defence system* that distracts from the existential anxieties associated with the uncertainty of sickness, pain and death, or the enormity of the task of dealing with it? The powerful denial of the cost of the consequences of the disruptions involved suggests that this might be so.

Menzies Lyth noted the resistance to change in the NHS of the 1950s and saw it as part of the social defence system of the time. But half a century on, it begins to look as if the pendulum has swung, and the uncritical acceptance and promotion of constant change in the NHS has taken its place.

Certainly, the approach to reorganisation tends to be simplistic, high on ideology, low on detail. There is little or no attempt to evaluate the *goodness of fit* between the new structure and the emotional task of caring for ill patients. Risk assessments working out the impact on the whole system are almost non-existent. Negative consequences are numerous because there is little attempt to foresee or pre-empt them. This evangelical approach could be interpreted as a manic defence that seeks to deny the complexity of providing healthcare to people who may suffer and die. There is a lack of understanding, a lack of thoughtful connection – a lack of kindness in the way the organisation as a whole is treated.

Thanks to the work of people like Goodall and Chance, anyone who intends to play around with the banana economy in a group of chimpanzees is responsible for the potential damage that can be done. Less scientifically, most of us are aware of the likely effects of approaching a hive of bees quietly getting on with its peaceful cooperative task and prodding it with a stick. The apparently ingrained denial, then, is more than obscuring the difficulty and limits involved in healthcare: it extends to a failure to attend to the destructive potential of change. It suggests a spiralling process of subjecting the NHS to unacknowledged anxiety, failure to notice its effects, and constantly growing recourse to 'omnipotent' manipulation. Concern about the financial cost of the NHS, its strengths and weaknesses, is inevitable and right. However, unless the powerful and persecutory anxiety evoked in society and government is acknowledged and better contained, the destructive spiral is set to continue. Therapeutic culture needs to be prioritised, to be allowed to develop. The conditions that evoke a hedonic culture need to be fostered and room allowed for them to bear fruit.

Divided loyalties, fragmented leadership

Another side-effect of inexorable structural change has been a proliferation of project managers, governance and improvement leads, initiative co-ordinators and 'champions'. The result is a confused and fragmented set of relationships and accountabilities. Hierarchies are complicated by many masters, all requiring satisfaction from front-line staff, and all offering the opportunity for endless displacement of power and responsibility. Leaders and managers find their sense of responsibility and authority diluted and blurred, as they attempt to answer to, and exercise their judgement in, this web of fragmented accountability. Menzies Lyth talked about the 'purposeful obscurity in the distribution of responsibility' (1988, p. 58) as a social defence against anxiety and, despite the rhetoric of flattened hierarchies, 'lean' organisations and performance management in the modern NHS, this phenomenon is as bad, or worse, than ever. A consequence is that problems in the ways things are done can become everybody's and nobody's business. As a result, crucial norms, and the relationships required to express them in action, are hard to build and trust.

This situation might improve if the role of 'operational manager' was more valued and strengthened. There is the real danger in many places that an 'up to the minute' focus on business efficiency leads to managers of business and improvement processes being more valued than leaders of the services that the organisation is there to provide. Added to this, rapid promotions mean operational managers tend to be moved on quickly, before they have accrued enough experience or developed the appropriate skills. This trend reflects a serious underestimation of the complexity of supporting good-quality care. It is worth considering whether *more* operational managers, all equipped with a wider range of skills, including business, psychosocial and 'improvement' skills, might not provide a more integrated and coherent leadership than the current mix.

The cost of overloading the system

Whatever the underlying driving forces are, it is clear that the constant changes have taken their toll on the workforce. There is anger that organisational change usually lacks an adequate evidence base (Oxman *et al*, 2005), that commitments are often rashly made to huge upheavals at huge cost in what are no more than experiments, with no one sure that innovation is going to result in something better. For clinicians trained in a system where the burden of proof is subject to exhaustive scientific rigour, this is particularly galling. Their trust in and commitment to the work of the service is consequently undermined.

The reorganisation which began in 2010 proceeded without public mandate, indeed counter to assurances given by the coalition government.

This absence, along with the fast pace and the underlying anxiety, feeds a culture of unsafety, and unreflective implementation. Change is experienced as being dogmatic, imposed from the top, poorly researched, understood and justified. Throughout the system there is the perception of clumsy implementation of policy without the mediation of intelligence and skill, implemented in a rush and frequently incompetently project managed. There is high anxiety that patient care will suffer. Add to this the history of the requirement for year-on-year efficiency savings, the reality of the financial crisis and wider public sector cuts and the stage is set for a messy process characterised by ugly conflict, power battles and scapegoating. The already high turnover of NHS trust chief executive officers is likely to continue. The average time in the job is usually quoted as 2–3 years and the proportion who are 'moved on' is very high. Any 'buffering' of the turmoil of change from the top of NHS organisations is weakened by such high turnover.

The Healthcare Commission highlights the fact that frequent changes at the top are detrimental to the functioning of trusts. It also observes that senior leaders are more likely to fail in organisations that are subject to particular external threats, such as forced mergers and reconfiguration of services, forced reorganisations and responsibility for substantial capital projects. After the outbreaks of *Clostridium difficile* that killed 33 people in Stoke Mandeville Hospital and 90 at the Maidstone and Tunbridge NHS Trust, the Healthcare Commission (2007) commented:

Both Trusts had undergone difficult mergers, were preoccupied with finance, and had a demanding agenda for reconfiguration and PFI [Private Finance Initiative], all of which consumed the time and effort of senior managers.

The conclusions of the inquiry into Mid-Staffordshire NHS Trust challenged these same priorities:

While structures are an important and necessary part of governance, what is really important is that they deliver the desired outcome, namely safe and good quality care. There is evidence that setting up systems predominated over improving actual outcomes for patients. (Francis, 2010, p. 398)

The fact that the majority of senior management time, including clinical management, is frequently focused on implementing structural change rather than on improving services is one of the reasons cited for disappointing rates of progress in some clinical areas. In Mid-Staffordshire, for example, the emergency admissions unit at the centre of the inquiry had been moved to different directorates three times between 2002 and 2007 and had had four different managers.

Lip service is often given within the service to the idea of *distributed leadership*, but there is little effort to involve front-line staff in planned change. At worst, this means there is little understanding of the rationale for change, let alone opportunity for teams to work through their feelings and adapt a centrally driven innovation to their local situation. Without the chance to develop a sense of ownership, staff will not commit themselves and their goodwill. Often the well-intentioned idea driving one initiative does not coordinate with the well-intentioned idea driving another initiative emanating from a different part of the organisation or Department of Health. Front-line staff feel caught in the conflict. There is often a sense that clinical staff are left accountable for keeping the service going whatever the unavoidable disruptive effects of the changes afoot.

Because of the frequent implementation of new initiatives within the NHS, most services will be going through a major change, recovering from a major change or preparing for a major change – and frequently all three at the same time. Sometimes change offers an opportunity to refocus on patients' experiences and needs as central to the task in a way that promotes kindness. Sometimes a shake-up of a team will bring unspoken conflicts and differences out into the open in a way that promotes kinder thinking on the part of staff members. But change, by definition, upsets the status quo and even when it is well managed and welcomed by staff it can distract from the primary task of caring for patients. While this can be mitigated to a degree by good operational leadership focused on helping staff to be mindful of the here-and-now task in hand, it is an uphill struggle when change is so frequent that the longed for period of stability never comes.

If therapeutic cultures are to re-form, there is an urgent need for integrated and *stable* leadership throughout the system. To develop the understanding and resources to address the forces tipping towards agonic or agonistic cultures requires relationships to be built, trust to be developed, confidence to grow. Difficulties in implementation and/or achieving outcomes need to be faced *as problems* requiring thought and work, rather than *as failures* requiring structural or personnel changes. Above all, leaders are required who can manage their anxiety – about performance, even survival – sufficiently to convey genuineness, readiness to face reality and compassion towards their staff.

Change and grief

The emotional response to change on the part of staff is frequently perceived and labelled as resistance, reaction or self-interest – an inconvenience. Bereavement evokes similar emotions, but tends not simply to be regarded as wilful inconvenience. Any change, especially imposed from 'outside', is emotionally disruptive and can affect the way people think about their work, their colleagues, their patients and themselves. Most staff are attached to their job and particular ways of working. They invest valued parts of themselves, often at personal cost, and take pride in what their particular service offers. They have found ways of managing their difficult feelings, ways that have become intimately entwined with the way things have been done. A culture where the focus is always on newness leaves people feeling insecure, undervalued and sometimes abandoned. If their service is cut or redesigned, they will feel bereaved, even if they can understand the reasons for the change.

Sometimes service changes come piling in so quickly on top of each other that staff involved in opening a new service will be required to close it only a few years – or even, in extreme cases, months – later. This can feel devastating, particularly for those who had responsibility for getting the service up and running. New services, like new babies, demand intense attention, especially where the quality of the service relies less on technology and more on people and developing a therapeutic psychosocial milieu. A service being cut dead before this aspiration has had a chance to mature and fulfil its promise can arouse feelings of loss that can be similar to bereavement. The present rate of change allows no time for helping staff work through appropriate grief for what has been lost. Indeed, the anxious drive towards change makes it hard to conceive of such feelings being natural and grieving people, if not regarded as resistant, will very likely be expected to move on immediately, to put in the extra effort required to start up a different role in the newly designed service.

Change and the organisational dynamic

Organisations and teams as a whole struggle with similar tensions as individuals. Change is always destabilising. Although it offers a chance to take a fresh look at habits that might have become institutionalised, explore new ways of working and implement improvements, in the process it risks stirring up old tensions and interfering with good practice. In an ideal situation, the ideas for the changes being implemented will have emerged from staff teams or chime well with changes they have been thinking about. Indeed, a well-run, well-functioning service will constantly be on the look-out for ways of improving its practice as it digests constructive feedback from patients and absorbs new guidelines or examples of best practice.

Even in this situation, though, the inevitable ambivalence and loss involved in change will be played out in the organisation and its constituent teams somehow, and needs attention. Most individuals actually have mixed feelings about change and are able to see advantages and disadvantages, particularly when the issue is something as complicated as the delivery of healthcare. It is, though, surprisingly difficult to hold on to mixed feelings in groups. There is always a tendency to polarise around a difficult issue rather than accommodate the uncertain middle ground. The result is often a team comprising an unproductive mix of: 'gung-ho' optimists, who proceed clumsily, without clarity about complexity or risk; die-hard conservatives, who resist without opening themselves to new thinking; and the disengaged, whose energy and intelligence are wasted. If such polarisation is not addressed, change may be more of an appearance than a reality, with old ways simply being packaged in new forms and results not reflecting the intentions behind the change. Problems of implementation frequently become personalised, with scapegoating and blame undermining group well-being and effectiveness.

People will be able to develop more nuanced views, and to find better ways of coping with and managing change, if leaders can resist the tendency to idealise the new and to denigrate the past. Allowing that there are good reasons for grief, because something valuable is being lost, and good reasons for scepticism about the new, because nothing is perfect, enables staff better to manage the group process involved in change.

Sensitive attention to the experience of staff will often, paradoxically, involve acknowledgement of the very disillusionment they feel. To face the reality that a previous way of working may have shortcomings is difficult, but people are more likely to commit to improving things if they have done so. If they see a cherished plan aborted, they may well be disillusioned with the leaders who instigate or allow its termination. Straightforward acknowledgement is much more effective than evangelical or coercive positive thinking – management attitudes that are as distressingly common as they are guaranteed to lower morale even further. Such a mature approach from senior management, of course, requires the capacity on their part, too, to manage anxiety – the anxiety that the staff will not cooperate, are incompetent or destructive, the anxiety that the organisation (and its managers) will fail.

Disillusion

Underneath the inevitable loss and disillusionment involved in change is a more disturbing *disillusionment*, particularly among senior clinicians and GPs. Reviewing and evaluating published complaints and criticisms of changes to the health service from medical doctors, Steve Iliffe, Professor of General Practice, emphasises 'the widespread discontent, the breadth and depth of feeling, and the entry into the argument of thoughtful and critical thinkers' (Iliffe, 2008, p. 4).

It is not uncommon to hear staff express a sense of being let down by the NHS:

My experience of colleagues who have given up general practice in recent years, blaming one or other aspect of the industrialisation of medicine, is that they did not lack commitment to the public health service, but did feel that it lacked commitment to them. (Iliffe, 2008, p. 3)

A loss of confidence in the NHS as an organisation that puts values into action through supporting valued staff in difficult work is very serious. Connection with the enterprise of kinship, with the social solidarity and commitment that the NHS represents, is undermined. It is as if a basic contract, an acknowledgement of interdependency, that underpins the expectation of commitment and generosity is at risk. The organisation depends on its staff taking on difficult responsibilities with commitment and skill, while individuals depend on the organisation to recognise their needs and support them with goodwill, compassion and intelligence. The capacity to 'hold' the anxiety of the work, to buffer the strain of continued effort and to support staff accordingly is crucial. If distrust of the organisation predominates, the capacity of staff to face the realities and complexities of patient need, to make the difficult decisions required and to act humanely inevitably suffers.

This is not an argument for complacency, for some heyday where staff could expect a job for life, and to be protected from the inconvenient complaints of patients. It is to stress the importance of people being able to trust each other to carry their share of the load of the responsibility and imagination for problem-solving. This is a scenario of collective interdependence, of mature relationships within which grown-ups can depend on each other, across roles and in the hierarchy, to work together to manage their tasks within a challenging and disrupted world. In *Managing Vulnerability*, Tim Dartington writes as follows:

A mature dependency is not, then, about the simple gratification of needs, passively demanded of an often absent leader. It is an interactive process, requiring both thought and action, where there is a recognition of difference and a use of difference to achieve mutually agreed ends. An aspect of dependency is therefore a capacity for followership, for responding to the leadership being offered in a purposeful way. (Dartington, 2010, p. 44)

If the basic contract to work together like this is at risk, especially in the way in which the processes and human costs of externally driven change are managed, the capacity for mutuality and kindness is fatally eroded. Andrew Cooper, Professor of Social Work, and Tim Dartington, writer and social scientist, considering the emotional life of contemporary organisations, comment on the weakening and increasing permeability of boundaries around organisations and what this means for the people involved (Cooper & Dartington, 2004). As the work organisation becomes increasingly unstable, it ceases to be experienced psychologically as a safe place and there is a consequent withdrawal of psychological investment. Cooper & Dartington describe a trend where employment becomes increasingly about survival only and 'environmentally blind individualism' is encouraged (p. 135).

Considering trends in private sector corporations, Susan Long, Professor of Creative and Sustainable Organisations at the Royal Melbourne Institute of Technology University, Australia, writes:

During times of rapid change, alongside the breakdown of many institutional values comes an increase in uncertainty and anxiety, a questioning of identity, disenchantment and pain. In recent years, this has led to a narcissistic defence against these feelings. Evidenced through isolation, withdrawal, instrumental attitudes to work and a sense of beating the system before it beats you. (Long, 2008, p. 157)

In these trends can be found the tilt towards the agonic mode, and the roots of worse – an agonistic world of conflict and brutality.

The nature of the problem goes further, though, than simply the way in which people and change are managed. The attempts to improve and reform the NHS reflect and embody ideologies and attitudes that profoundly colour the 'organisation in the mind' (Armstrong, 2005). In themselves – and especially when they are poorly managed – they tend to pull the work away from applied kinship, from attentive kindness to patients as people, towards instrumentality, towards mechanical behaviour, even towards neglect and active abuse.

References

Armstrong, D. (2005) *Organisation in the Mind: Psychoanalysis, Group Relations and Organizational Consultancy*. Karnac.

Blair, T. (2000) Quoted in C. Webster (2002) *The National Health Service: A Political History*. Oxford University Press, p. 238.

Chance, M. R. A. (1988) *Social Fabrics of the Mind*. Lawrence Erlbaum Associates.

Cooper, A. & Dartington, T. (2004) The vanishing organization. In *Working Below the Surface* (eds C. Huffington, D. Armstrong, W. Halton, *et al*), pp. 127–150. Karnac.

Dartington, T. (2010) *Managing Vulnerability: The Underlying Dynamics of Systems of Care*. Karnac.

Department of Health (2000) *The NHS Plan*. HMSO.

Department of Health (2010) *Equity and Excellence: Liberating the NHS*. Available at http://www. dh.gov.uk/en/Publicationsandstatistics/Publications/PublicationsPolicyAndGuidance/ DH_117353 (last accessed March 2011).

Francis, R. (2010) *The Independent Inquiry into Care Provided by Mid-Staffordshire NHS Foundation Trust, January 2005–March 2009*. HMSO.

Goodall, J. (1965) Chimpanzees of the Gombe Stream Reserve. In *Primate Behaviour* (ed. I. DeVore), pp. 425–473. Holt, Rinehart and Winston.

Ham, C. (2009) Lessons from the past decade for future health reforms. *BMJ*, **339**, b4372.

Healthcare Commission (2007) *The Investigation Report into* Clostridium difficile *at Maidstone and Tunbridge Wells NHS Trust*. HMSO.

Hirschhorn, L. (1988) *The Workplace Within: Psychodynamics of Organisational Life*. MIT Press.

HM Government (2010) *The Coalition: Our Programme for Government*. Cabinet Office. Available at http://www.cabinetoffice.gov.uk/media/409088/pfg_coalition.pdf (last accessed March 2011).

Iliffe, S. (2008) *From General Practice to Primary Care: The Industrialization of Family Medicine*, Oxford University Press.

Long, S. (2008) *The Perverse Organisation and Its Deadly Sins*. Karnac.

Menzies Lyth, I. (1959) The functions of social systems as a defence against anxiety: a report on a study of the nursing service of a general hospital. *Human Relations*, **13**, 95–121. Reprinted in I. Menzies Lyth (1988) *Containing Anxiety in Institutions: Selected Essays, Vol. I*, pp. 43–88. Free Association Books.

National Audit Office (2010) *Reorganising Central Government*. HMSO.

Oxman, A., Sackett, D., Chalmers, I., *et al* (2005) A surrealistic meta-analysis of redisorganisation theories. *Journal of the Royal Society of Medicine*, **98**, 563–568.

Power, M. D. (1988) The cohesive foragers: human and chimpanzee. In *Social Fabrics of the Mind* (ed. M. R. A. Chance), pp. 75–104. Lawrence Erlbaum Associates.

Smith, J., Walshe, K. & Hunter, D. (2001) The redisorganisation of the NHS. (Editorial.) *BMJ*, **323**, 1262–1263.

Walshe, K. (2010) Reorganisation of the NHS in England. (Editorial.) *BMJ*, **341**, c3843.

CHAPTER 10

The pull towards perversion

So are they all, all honourable men....
(Shakespeare, *Julius Caesar*)

Perverse dynamics

The health service sits within a broader society that shapes its rules, agreements and unconscious social pacts. In the Introduction, we noted the spirit of cooperation that was around in the immediate aftermath of the Second World War and how this provided the value base and a fertile ground for implementing the welfare state. There is little doubt, though, that such communalism has been steadily encroached upon by individualism, consumerism, acquisition and exploitation, even greed, since then. What sort of organisations do *these* values nurture?

Susan Long attempts to answer this in her book *The Perverse Organisation and Its Deadly Sins*. A basic premise of her book is that there has been a move in society generally from a culture of *narcissism* (Lasch, 1979) to elements of a culture of *perversion* (Long, 2008, p. 1). Perversion flourishes where *instrumental* relations have dominance – in other words, where people are used as a means to an end, as tools and commodities rather than respected citizens. It is these relations that Long sees predominating increasingly. Her book considers large private corporations rather than the public sector. However, the fashion to idealise large private sector corporations and the subsequent corporatisation of the public sector means much of the thinking in her book is relevant to the modern NHS.

Perversion is not simply a deviation from normative morality, or occasional failures in the healthy struggle with mixed feelings described in earlier chapters. Perversion is about seeking individual gain and pleasure at the expense of the common good, often to the extent of not recognising the existence of others or their rights. For many people, the word conjures up extreme examples, such as the sadistic murderer Harold Shipman, or the appalling stories of physically and sexually abusive teachers and priests that hit the headlines regularly: a world everyone would prefer to distance themselves from.

Perversion may seem a strong word to associate with the health service. But it does capture some of the internal contradictions and destructive dynamics at work that draw cynicism and worse out of the most well intentioned, hard-working staff member. It is well to remember that perverse individuals and organisations do not see themselves as such and many of them appear to others as 'kind'. By all accounts, Dr Shipman had all the characteristics of a good GP. He gave the impression of 'being kind and avuncular and of working tirelessly for his patients', while in fact being a prolific serial killer (Barkham, 2002). A fundamental aspect of perversion is the process of *turning a blind eye* and, with this, the development of perverse certainty, the denial of a reality that continues to be encountered and the consequent self-deception that seduces accomplices and breeds corruption.

It is important to realise that Long's emphasis is on perversity displayed by institutions, rather than by their leaders or members. There is no suggestion that individual NHS workers, as people, are any more perverse than workers in any other organisation. Nevertheless, in reality, an organisation and its members are entwined: the decisions and actions of individuals are influenced by organisational culture, and, in turn, reinforce it, for good or ill. The concept of perversion sheds light on frankly exploitative behaviour, helps explain how many people in positions of trust end up abusing those positions and how people may be collectively perverse despite individual attempts to be otherwise. Can the use of this term be justified when the NHS is considered?

Knowing and not knowing

It is always difficult for those involved at the time to understand the macro-changes in the culture of which they are part. For this reason, Steve Iliffe appeals to his readers to engage with these issues and make 'social reality legible to ourselves and our communities' (Iliffe, 2008, p. 203). Knowing and not knowing at one and the same time is central to the concept of perversion.

There appear to be powerful forces working against making the social reality of the NHS 'legible'. These forces, indeed, seem often to be striving actively to prevent acknowledgement of problems, especially where they may be consequences of key elements of the 'reform agenda' of whatever government is in power. This force can show itself in relatively undramatic ways. Managers and leaders, convinced about the benefits of (or dependent for their success on) one change or another, may simply minimise the evidence of problems or of unintended consequences. They may try to persuade staff who see problems that they are being negative and overlook the costs to them and the service. Such behaviour, in itself, undermines confidence and common purpose.

But there are far more serious – and quite explicitly perverse and corrupting – manifestations of this enforced 'blind eye'. In Mid-Staffordshire NHS Foundation Trust between 2005 and 2009, an estimated 400–1200 people attending through the emergency department died as a result of cost-cutting, target-driven behaviour and poor management. A report by the Healthcare Commission concluded:

In the Trust's drive to become a foundation trust, it appears to have lost sight of its real priorities. The Trust was galvanised into radical action by the imperative to save money and did not properly consider the effect of reductions in staff on the quality of care. It took a decision to significantly reduce staff without adequately assessing the consequences. Its strategic focus was on financial and business matters at a time when the quality of care of its patients admitted as emergency was well below acceptable standards. (Healthcare Commission, 2009, p. 11)

These statements, although they describe the danger of unmitigated financial efficiency drives, overlook a far more sinister process. The trust *knew* about these dangers and of the increasingly obvious effects. Managers and leaders appear to have ignored, or even silenced, feedback from staff at all levels that would have alerted them to the problem. Staff tried – more than a third of the 515 safety incident reports submitted by ward staff attributed the problem to inadequate staffing. Consultants found their incident reports downgraded to being minor events without consultation or investigation. One senior consultant used parliamentary privilege to expose this climate to the Parliamentary Health Select Committee. Despite the enormous attention given over the past decade to clinical governance systems, reporting – far from helping the trust manage the quality of its services – lost credibility completely. A senior manager in the trust even called for a specialist independent investigator to remove any statements in his report suggesting that people had died because of poor care – because it would distress people and bring bad publicity for the trust (Francis, 2010, p. 23). This story illustrates directly what is meant by the 'pull towards perversion'.

In fact, this illustration captures a wider landscape in which this 'knowing and not knowing' is growing in its grip. Tony Delamothe, Deputy Editor of the *BMJ*, contrasted the attention and public awareness relating to a range of earlier 'scandals', such as Alder Hey, Bristol Children's Heart Surgery, and Harold Shipman, with more recent inquiries, such as those into deaths through hospital infection in several trusts, and the Mid-Staffordshire case itself (Delamothe, 2010). He argued that there appeared to be a determination to regard recent scandals as rare exceptions, and to fail to note patterns – despite the apparent consistency and frequency of examples of similar concerns. He comments that there 'should be enough material for a meta-inquiry into English medical scandals of the 21st Century'. It appears that there is active resistance to what is 'known' being directly acknowledged and made properly available for understanding and action. This resistance is at the core of the 'pull towards perversion'.

Corrupting forces?

There appear to be three closely intertwined processes at work. None of them is perverse in itself – but separately and together they can create perverse dynamics in the context of healthcare. The first is the active promotion of a competitive market economy, on the basis of a commodified view of need, skills and service. Such an economy works against the idea of an integrated service that prioritises the needs of vulnerable patients, and can insidiously affect the attitudes, feelings and relationships of staff. The second is the process of industrialising healthcare. This enterprise has the potential to undermine healthcare as work undertaken by skilled individuals in relationships with patients and to turn it into the mechanical delivery of processes and systems. The third is the framework and currency of specification, regulation and performance management. How services are specified, monitored and evaluated – and funded – has a profound effect on the day-to-day clinical work.

These three elements are of course interrelated and, some would say, reflect trends in society at large. But of particular concern is the way these processes have taken hold without proper debate and understanding. It is crucial that the potential of these processes to skew, even actively pervert, the delivery of healthcare is recognised and managed.

The increasing uncritical predominance of the market paradigm is the dangerous growing medium for a range of perverse attitudes and behaviours that pull attention and commitment away from kinship and kindness at best, and lead to a range of active abuses at worst. This is not a simple matter of debating whether healthcare delivery should be through a 'mixed economy' of public, third-sector and private organisations. A market-based approach influences how every part of the system – patient, illness, staff member, treatment, location of treatment and so on – is valued, defined and treated. It is founded in a worldview of commodities, competing technologies and providers, customers and prices.

Crowding out altruism

People become commodities, valued for their place in the market rather than their intrinsic worth. At the same time, economic rationalism has affected us all, with the imperative to make money increasingly valued more than the intrinsic value of work. In the 2009 BBC Reith Lectures, Michael Sandel argued the importance of a politics orientated less to the pursuit of individual self-interest and more to the pursuit of the common good (Sandel, 2009a,b). He was critical of the market triumphalism of the past three decades, particularly the expansion of markets into new social problem areas such as prisons and healthcare. In a highly pertinent and important turn of phrase, he said we were 'drifting from having a market economy to becoming a market society'. In other words, rather than holding on to a sense that we have collectively *constructed* a market better to organise aspects of our creative, entrepreneurial, trading and economic life, we have now begun to *think and define* ourselves and everything else in terms of market values.

An important part of Sandel's critique is the belief that markets are not neutral or inert. The move of markets and market thinking into social areas previously governed by non-market norms actually shifts these norms in a way that may be undesirable. A classic study in this field looked at different systems of blood donation (Titmuss, 1971). It compared the US system, which permitted the buying and selling of blood for transfusion, with the UK system, which relied wholly on voluntarily donated blood and banned financial incentives. To the surprise of some, the commercialisation of blood in the USA led to shortages, inefficiencies and a greater incidence of contaminated blood. Titmuss concluded that putting a price on blood had turned what had been a gift into a commodity: once blood is bought and sold in the marketplace, people are less likely to feel a moral obligation to donate out of altruism. Introducing a market value eroded the non-market norms – the norms of kinship and kindness – associated with blood donation, with very serious effects.

As further evidence that markets leave their mark on social values, Sandel talked about a child care centre where the parents were routinely turning up late at the end of the day with the result that centre staff had to stay on longer than they wished. They decided to start charging fees for lateness, expecting this to act as a disincentive, with the hope that staff could go home on time. To their surprise, it had the opposite effect and the number of late pick-ups increased. Parents seemed to find that paying for the extra time removed the anxiety and guilt and entitled them to be late. In this example, what was intended as a fine for 'bad' parents became a fee for a commodity. Parents stopped worrying about being late for their children and decided it was a service worth paying for. Attaching a financial tariff to lateness changed it into something else and altered the thinking and behaviour of the parents (Sandel, 2009a, p. 7).

Topical in Britain in 2009 was a debate about the definition of illegal child-minding. Two women who arranged their work shifts so that they could look after each other's children had been told they were breaking the law because neither of them was a registered child-minder, and they were ordered to send the children to nursery. The issue centred on the concept of reward (framed by OFSTED in completely financial terms) despite the fact that no money changed hands. The public were at first reassured that it is acceptable to look after each other's children providing it is for no more than 2 hours, no more than 14 days per year! It seems that the law could no longer accept that one might help out another parent from a sense of mutuality, fondness and enjoyment of their children, and, indeed, kindness. In the end, a government minister stepped in and overruled the OFSTED guidelines, but the whole sorry episode shows how close we are to becoming a society where helping each other out can be seen only as the regulated trade of a commodity for gain.

Commodification, then, poses a direct threat to a culture of kinship, responsibility to each other, and kindness. However important it is to be able to relate cost to task in healthcare, this danger requires serious attention.

An economy of kindness?

Many economists would claim that a monetary value can be put on anything and that attributing a market price to something like 'happiness' enables us to measure social progress in ways that do not rely only on measures of production and consumption. By putting market prices on two very different things, one has, in theory, a way of comparing their relative value and weighing one against the other. This is the theory behind the area of health service research that tries to evaluate and compare the quality of life achieved rather than just survival rates. There are, for example, measures of quality-adjusted life years (QALYs) and disability-adjusted life years (DALYs) that have been developed to help balance the benefits of particular treatments for various conditions or even to weigh up the value of keeping someone with a terminal, or severe chronic, condition alive. The problem comes in deciding how to set about putting a value on life in its various guises. Highly technical cost–benefit analyses have been developed with their own internal logic, but this is controversial and ultimately somewhat random, as a recent example cited in a *BMJ* editorial exemplifies:

The National Institute for Health and Clinical Excellence (NICE) requires strong reasons for supporting an intervention that costs more than £30,000 ($49,200) to deliver a year of good quality life. The Department of Transport generally puts a much higher value on life when deciding on measures to reduce the risk of road and rail deaths. This implies that lives could be saved with no extra overall expenditure by diverting resources from spending on road and rail safety to spending on medical interventions. (Weale, 2009)

Needless to say, the author was not proposing this as a policy, but using it to illustrate the difficulties inherent in attributing a monetary cost to the value of life and the wide discrepancy between models used in different government departments. In his final Reith Lecture, Sandel showed up the absurdity of what he called 'market mimicking governance'. He gave the example of a cost–benefit analysis of new air pollution standards done a few years ago by the US Environmental Protection Agency, where it assigned a monetary value to human life: $3.7 million per life saved, except for people over the age of 70, whose lives were valued at $2.3 million. Sandel went on:

Lying behind the different valuations, was a market-mimicking assumption: younger people, with more years still to live, would presumably pay more to save their lives than older people would pay to save theirs. Advocates for the elderly didn't see it that way. They bitterly protested the 'senior citizen discount!' (Sandel, 2009*b*)

Sandel sees the idea that everything can be captured in monetary terms as seductive because it offers a way of making political choices without making hard and controversial moral decisions. The problem starts when cost–benefit analysis is treated as if it were a science rather than a subjective conceptual model. Monetary valuations, and the process of internal logic through which they are derived, become imbued with much more significance than is sensible. This shifts decision-making from the realm of democratic politics concerned with the common good, to 'experts' responsible for a technical tool – what Sandel describes as an 'ultimately spurious science'. This spurious science appears to have found rather too many uncritical students among commissioners and contract managers.

The problems arise when economic measures become idealised as 'objective', prioritised over other equally valid measures, and used to duck bigger social and ethical decisions. Commissioning, research and even clinical protocols then get skewed. The real danger comes when people start to think that recovery from, for example, depression *equates* to and can be *assessed in terms of* economic recovery, and that services that *prioritise* such recovery are most important. In fact, depression is a condition that affects our mood, thoughts and relationships, the improvement of which many would rate as more important than the capacity to function at work.

This progression – from a useful economic model to an idea that gets built into social transactions in a way that affects the way we think about ourselves and each other – is what Sandel means when he talks about moving from *having* a market economy to *being* a market society. We increasingly find ourselves thinking in terms of the monetary cost or value of things in a way that crowds out other meanings. The uncritical substitution of economic measures for political, moral and ethical judgement fractures the bond between us as human beings sharing a difficult world. It removes the person from the picture – and without the person it is hard to stay connected to kinship and kindness.

Sandel illuminates this issue by considering a proposal that is pertinent to the concept of kindness when he takes up a 'brainwave' by an unnamed American academic for solving the question of asylum seekers. The idea this thinker had advanced was that an international body should assign each country a yearly refugee quota, based on national wealth, and then let nations buy and sell among themselves. According to standard market logic this policy could prove efficient and benefit all involved, but Sandel reflects on his distaste with the idea:

What exactly is objectionable about it? It has something to do with the fact that a market in refugees changes our view of who refugees are and how they should be treated. It encourages the participants – the buyers, the sellers and also those whose asylum is being haggled over – to think of refugees as burdens to be unloaded or as revenue sources rather than human beings in peril. (p. 6)

145

The commodification of vocation

The concept of vocation is useful here. Vocation literally means 'calling', the implication being that one has been called by some destiny or God to follow a certain path. For the religious, this links to the concept of 'grace', a gift or help coming from God. This idea – religious or secular – has been a source of energy for many generations of professionals. Although most people today would interpret vocation in a less literal way, it continues to convey a sense that one's chosen profession is more than just a job. It suggests that one is deeply privileged to have the opportunity and the expertise to be involved in healthcare. It leads to an active welcoming of the responsibilities and duties involved that goes beyond the detail of a job plan or financial reward. This may seem old fashioned, not to mention open to abuse. However, throughout the NHS, from secretary to chief executive, there are still thousands of staff who would subscribe to such an attitude, and who commit themselves to their work inspired by such feelings.

There is a real worry that the introduction of a more commercial paradigm has done more harm than good. *Commodifying* the work of professionals has undermined the intrinsic value, satisfaction and enjoyment of that work, and threatens dangerously to undermine the concept of vocation to serve. For patients, always searching for signs that the professional really cares, this is bad news.

Over the first decade of the century, NHS staff were subject to a new consultant contract, the general medical services contract for GPs and 'Agenda for Change' – a framework for the pay grades and career development for non-medical staff (all available at http://www.dh.gov.uk). These are all attempts to make expectations more explicit and equitable, and pay more transparent and fair. While many staff benefited financially (particularly the better-paid) there was a general sense among clinicians that the initiatives caused dissatisfaction and worsened morale. Medical consultants, for example, were promised the contract would enable them to be paid for what they actually did and the hours they actually worked. In the attempt to create equity, they had to account for every hour of their time using diaries and fit the described activity into bureaucratic categories. Anything over and above the standard job description had to be haggled for. Prior to this, the informal understanding was that they were paid to do their appointed job with whatever it took in terms of extra hours.

Unfortunately, there had been a gross underestimation of what the new scheme would actually cost – based in part on the suspicion that doctors were doing far less for the NHS than they were. Trusts were forced to look for opportunities to save money and limit the number of consultant sessions it would allow people to do – or, indeed, to cut back on other services to fund the gap. Many consultants continue to work well above the 40-hour working week, despite being contracted for less. Most of them are better paid than they were before the contract (National Audit Office,

2007). But the sense of grievance is higher because there is now a system that purports to pay them by the session rather than emphasising their responsibility and trusting them to get on and do the job. They have been encouraged to count their hours and think of their time at work in terms of units of pay. Moreover, the activity during these contracted sessions has been defined in detail, which leads to a sense that anything over and above this cannot be recognised by the system. Often it is activity over and above what is expected that brings job satisfaction and is important to patients. In job-planning meetings, however, the consultant and manager often end up haggling over which activity should be dropped.

Sometimes it is possible to concentrate instead on the integral value of the work, recognising and affirming pride in achievements. Such meetings proceed very differently and consultants may well leave poorer but happier – or happier until they start chatting to colleagues, comparing workload and pay and reverting to a 'counting the cost' mentality! There are worries that linking the job in such detail to financial rewards encroaches upon the values that have traditionally driven consultants. Put more crudely, doctors did not tend to see themselves as 'wage slaves' until recently.

Incentive packages for GPs have been around since 1990, when the first new contract sought to incentivise health promotion by identifying patients at risk. The 2004 contract implemented a fresh approach to this, by micro-managing consultations in selected clinical areas through a complex system of targets. The effectiveness of such measures for improving the quality of clinical care is still undetermined. The impact of shifting the balance from autonomy towards prescription for practitioners requires consideration. The consequences of focusing on narrow areas of need for thinking about the whole person and whole system have yet to be fully understood. One obvious lesson is that incentives need to be seen by GPs as important to clinical practice if they are to succeed. In general, if economic factors outweigh professional imperatives there are risks to the NHS of doctors and other professionals 'gaming' the system – a phenomenon that has to indicate a cynicism and halfheartedness that is likely to rub off on patients (Iliffe, 2008, p. 96).

'Agenda for Change' was introduced in 2005 and is basically a pay scale system tied into a knowledge and skills framework covering all NHS staff apart from doctors and top managers. Staff moving on to this system had to fill in an extremely long form giving details of their work, which was then scored under various domains such as physical strain, emotional pressure, concentration and responsibility. Just like the consultant contract, the new system was far more problematic than anticipated by policy-makers, and ended up costing far more money. But of concern is how much, and in what way, it affected the values that drive the work of the NHS. At the time, there was a strong sense of a process similar to those Sandel considers. Staff were being encouraged (often, but not always, accidently) to describe – and in some cases, indeed, to exaggerate – the *burdensome* nature of their job in order to be banded and paid as highly as possible.

These approaches to defining healthcare tasks, and to remunerating work, have resulted in unhealthy levels of competitiveness and envy. Most worryingly, they have encouraged a negative way of thinking about the job that focuses on onerous tasks rather than the relationship with patients. They have pushed the experience of caring for the sick in the direction of the model for caring for refugees that so concerned Sandel – except the 'haggling' over the burden and reward is not between nations but between professions and individual staff members. Staff are drawn towards *trading their skills* rather than *valuing them in terms of how they serve the patient*.

This process of commodification of healthcare, and the subsequent promotion of competition in relation to burden and remuneration, has introduced a market into the heart of NHS services – no less real than the wider competitive market promoted by New Labour and in the coalition White Paper *Equity and Excellence: Liberating the NHS* (Department of Health, 2010). It is one of the forces that, unexamined and unmanaged, pulls towards the perversion of care.

The NHS market

There have been numerous steps in the introduction of a market philosophy to the health service in the past three decades, starting with the Griffiths report in 1983 and resulting in the incremental and confusing process of putting in place the 'purchaser–provider' split, and, more recently, promoting a 'mixed economy of care'. The purchaser–provider split aims to build more accountability into the work of NHS providers, both for what they do and for how they spend money. It is intended to enable changes for the better in systems that might otherwise be rigid and resistant. Promoting a variety of providers has been seen as a way of fostering innovation, getting value for money and bolstering the capacity of existing services, through a competitive market. Whatever the merits of these ideas, they have been ideal vehicles for the steady importation of the ideology of a primitive kind of market competition, even of 'survival of the cheapest', into the NHS.

This process has been consciously driven in many cases, but has also increased in power as an unintended consequence of other aspects of the way the NHS is funded, evaluated and managed. The focus has steadily moved to the cost of defined processes and transactions, with a relatively undeveloped 'quality' component. The theory is that commissioners (the purchasers) will develop detailed specifications for what they want, build them into contracts and 'tender them out' to find someone to do them well at the cheapest price. Providers will be encouraged to become innovative, lean and efficient by the resulting competition. The whole system is predicated on the idea that the purchasers can specify well and also make accurate comparisons between offerings, and that there is a level playing field for providers. The approach relies on market-driven changes being managed well. And the idea that competition always promotes improvement.

Whether or not such conditions actually ever exist, the competitive dimension has been problematic. Different providers can apportion cost differently to the same processes, or claim, in ways specifications are too blunt to catch, that they can do the same things at a lower price. If an NHS provider loses the contract for a specific service (whether because of poor quality or higher cost), its ability to continue with its wider remit and services may be undermined. The concept of an integrated, universal service then suffers. A successful bidder for one aspect of healthcare may take on no responsibility for integrating that into the wider picture, with a similar result.

It is difficult to avoid the fact that the behaviour of some of the supposed 'partner' organisations in the market that now benefit from NHS money fulfils many of the criteria for perversion. For instance, it is common practice for large private companies to run a new project at a loss to start with. They can then outbid other providers, including the NHS, only to put up their costs to a commercial rate once the new service is established and the commissioners (and patients) have been hooked. Another example is the behaviour of private companies, often venture capitalists or large conglomerates investing in care homes for the elderly, selling off homes to make a quick profit when prices in the neighbourhood go up, despite the detrimental effect on the elderly residents in their care (Pollock, 2004, p. 180). The current expansion of the NHS foundation trust sector, though the underlying idea is often framed as that of social enterprise, means that the effects of the profit motive in this 'market' need careful watching.

The idea of healthcare as a marketed and purchased commodity seems to be increasing. It has been interesting (and infuriating) to see – on billboards, in leisure centres, in the media – advertisements for private healthcare putting forward as major benefits ways of working and services that are, in fact, commonplace and free through the NHS. Presumably, their marketing people think that citizens either do not know that, or are persuadable to purchase it as a style statement. The reality might be both or either. Another unpalatable aspect of some healthcare for profit is the incentive to sell care of questionable value to paying 'customers' – often people who would have been advised against treatment by dispassionate clinicians, or given a more comprehensive picture of the risks and implications.

Even without such frankly perverse activity, the involvement of the private sector, whatever its benefits, has been increasingly characterised by the contracting out of specific activities and treatments, with consequent fragmentation of the patient's care. The 2011 Health and Social Services Bill takes this to another level, by opening all services to 'any willing provider' – making the NHS into a market into which businesses can seek to enter, whatever their ethic, whatever their view of what justifies profit.

With increased competition and continued real-terms reductions in the funding of NHS services, there is a real danger of a vicious circle, making *integrated, universal healthcare* – the realisation of kinship – a lost aspiration.

There is conflicting evidence as to the effectiveness of competition in driving up quality. A lot has to do with how one defines and measures either of these categories, with some evidence of both positive and negative links (Propper *et al*, 2003, 2005; Cooper *et al*, 2010). Researchers raise strong caveats regarding the proposition that competition has a positive effect on the development of institutions. They also point out that payer-driven competition (commissioning) is not the same as competition promoted by patient choice. They imply that commissioners looking for cost savings may well be at odds with patients (however poorly or well informed) looking for choice. Most importantly, Propper and colleagues observe that a fixed-price system and a competitive market

gives hospitals incentives not to accept more severely ill patients ('dumping'), to undertreat such patients ('skimping') and to attract the less severely ill and overtreat these ('creaming') ... these incentives ... are intensified when hospitals are subject to actual competition or competition based on league tables. (Propper *et al*, 2005, p. 15)

This research – and a great deal of informed concern – points to the need for real caution, and much more understanding of the incentives and outcomes generated by competition. It is clear that a simple hedonic culture may lack the vigour and ambition to address the kinds of challenges faced in healthcare – that some creative competition for excellence and innovation may be required. However, the results of the Gombe experiment reported in the last chapter, where stimulating competition for bananas tipped a placid society over into brutality and murder, should be borne firmly in mind. 'Dumping', 'skimping', and 'creaming', as behaviours of institutions, look very much like a system moving towards brutality. Simplistic or ill-considered mimicry of markets in commodities is dangerous in healthcare, and a potential engine for perverting its delivery.

Internalising the market

The research, and the political debate, about competition is based on very short-term analysis, within a shifting frame of variously narrow measures. What it does not illuminate are the effects on the attitudes and work of staff within healthcare organisations. Such research is urgently needed. Whatever the problems with competition at institutional levels, it appears to have inexorably entered the culture of NHS organisations and into the minds of their staff. It smoulders there as a kind of destabilising anxiety, whether or not actual competitive tendering is happening. This anxiety is amplified in many cases by mistrust between commissioning staff and providers, and by poor management of the issue inside trusts. The anxiety, and the associated behaviours evoked, have rarely appeared to promote innovation and imagination, especially when allied to the unmanaged invasion of people's thinking and language by the 'cost for commodity' aspect of the market. The quest to 'do more for less', in the context of obscure competitive threats, has a corrosive effect.

Costing healthcare, seeking efficiency and improved performance are unavoidable, of course, and very difficult in a universal service or in the case of complex care or long-term conditions. But, partly because of the poor 'fit' between costing models and the reality of care, and partly because of the unfiltered injection of preoccupation with cost, activity and competition into organisations and their people, a dangerous process has occurred. Instead of being technical issues managed by management and business staff, they have profoundly coloured the daily life of healthcare provision.

All NHS staff are now aware of the contracts that define and sometimes restrict the work they do. They know that if their unit does not achieve the activity levels agreed (for good or bad reasons) or, indeed, if the commissioners simply choose to change the contract, there will be financial penalties and possible job losses. The consequent anxiety frequently invades the clinical relationship, with patients and with other services, and can skew practice. The degree of damage done is often amplified by the frequent disconnection between funding, contracting and specification and the realities of providing care and treatment.

Everywhere, staff face 'efficiency savings'. Although a few of these measures are well thought through and reflect genuine examination of the most efficient ways of meeting patient need, many are apportioned relatively blindly, with any mitigating service remodelling happening after the decision to cut. Any goodwill on the part of staff is undermined by the relentless, year-on-year and frequently unconsidered nature of this process. Even if subjecting healthcare to market forces were to be advisable, any belief that there is any rational 'market' at work would be fatally undermined by this financially driven, rather than value-driven, process. The process of increasing efficiency within limited resources is hard enough: being required to continue to deliver to specification whatever the funding reduction and setting out on unstable wheels into a competitive market at the same time can be crippling.

Caught between attention to the patient, and the contradictory and unpredictable demands of efficiency and pressure to provide poorly specified activity, clinical decisions in these situations are made by staff who have varying degrees of awareness that patients' welfare is not the priority. Many are distressed by their complicity with compromise. The nursing press, for example, has frequent articles and letters from nurses protesting about the poor quality of care they are involved in delivering (e.g. Maben *et al*, 2007). Other nurse authors have described colleagues as being 'deeply distressed at their perceived failure at meeting their patients' needs' (Chambers & Ryder, 2009, p. 53) or suffering 'moral distress' when their capacity to provide effective and compassionate care is limited by resources (Fournier *et al*, 2007, p. 262). It is common for clinical staff to feel a sense of frustration arising from their diminishing power to influence these systems while being increasingly made responsible both for making the system work and for patient care and outcome, when sometimes the two are contradictory.

Increasingly, staff find themselves thinking a sort of 'doublespeak' and, rather than live in a state of exhausting cognitive dissonance, they withdraw emotionally, become depressed or adopt a more cynical approach to the work. These are all ways of managing that inevitably undermine their capacity for kindness. Of more concern, though, is the pull into a perverse state of mind where the contradictions are denied and the erosion of values is unacknowledged and largely unconscious.

The unbuffered injection of anxiety, competition and preoccupation with activity and money into clinical services represents a dangerous threat to effective kindness. Whether the processes and policies that evoke these feelings are right or inevitable, ways of acknowledging and managing them, and ways of ensuring that the priority to serve the patient can remain uppermost in the minds of staff, are urgently required. While finding new ways of working, to improve both quality and efficiency, is important, it is also vital to find a way of ensuring that a 'more for less' mentality does not ignore the limits of the finite and pressurised resource that is those staff.

The potential of commodification of care, and the introduction of a market in it, fatally to undermine kinship and kindness requires at the very least recognition, not denial, and intelligent management, not cynicism. To address these tasks, it is important to understand the effects of two other closely related processes: the industrialisation of healthcare, and its regulation and performance management. It is these issues we consider in our next chapters.

References

Barkham, P. (2002) The Shipman report. *The Times*, 20 July, p. 15.

Chambers, C. & Ryder, E. (2009) *Compassion and Caring in Nursing*. Radcliffe.

Cooper, Z., Gibbons, S., Jones, S., *et al* (2010) *Does Hospital Competition Save Lives? Evidence from the English Patient Choice Reforms*. London School of Economics.

Delamothe, T. (2010) Repeat after me: 'Mid Staffordshire'. *BMJ*, **340**, c188.

Department of Health (2010) *Equity and Excellence: Liberating the NHS*. Available at http://www.dh.gov.uk/en/Publicationsandstatistics/Publications/PublicationsPolicyAndGuidance/DH_117353 (last accessed March 2011).

Fournier, B., Kipp, W. & Mill, J. (2007) The nursing care of AIDS patients in Uganda. *Journal of Transcultural Nursing*, **18**, 257–264.

Francis, R. (2010) *The Independent Inquiry into Care Provided by Mid-Staffordshire NHS Foundation Trust, January 2005–March 2009*. HMSO.

Griffiths, R. (1983) *Report of the NHS Management Inquiry*. HMSO.

Healthcare Commission (2009) *The Investigation into Mid Staffordshire NHS Foundation Trust*. Healthcare Commission.

Iliffe, S. (2008) *From General Practice to Primary Care: The Industrialization of Family Medicine*, Oxford University Press.

Lasch, C. (1979) *The Culture of Narcissism*. W. W. Norton.

Long, S. (2008) *The Perverse Organisation and Its Deadly Sins*. Karnac.

Maben, J., Latter, S. & Macleod Clark, J. (2007) The sustainability of ideals, values and the nursing mandate: evidence from a longitudinal qualitative study. *Nursing Enquiry*, **14**, 99–113.

National Audit Office (2007) *Pay Modernisation: A New Contract for NHS Consultants in England*. HMSO

Pollock, A. (2004) *NHS plc: The Privatization of Health Care*. Verso.

Propper, C., Burgess, S. & Gossage, D. (2003) *Competition and Quality: Evidence from the NHS Internal Market 1991–1999*. CMPO, University of Bristol.

Propper, C., Wilson, D. & Burgess, S. (2005) *Extending Choice in English Health Care: The Implications of the Economic Evidence*. CMPO, University of Bristol.

Sandel, M. (2009a) The Reith Lectures 2009, Lecture 1: 'Markets and morals', broadcast 9 June, BBC Radio 4.

Sandel, M. (2009b) The Reith Lectures 2009, Lecture 4: 'A new politics of the common good', broadcast 30 June, BBC Radio 4.

Titmuss, R. (1971) *The Gift Relationship: From Human Blood to Social Policy*. Reissued LSE Publications, eds A. Oakley & J. Ashton (1997).

Weale, M. (2009) Economic progress and health improvement. *BMJ*, **339**, 1097.

CHAPTER 11

Free to serve the public

Ordered to be kind, we are likely to be cruel; wanting to be kind, we are likely to discover our generosity. (Philips & Taylor, 2009, p. 52)

Two ways of seeing

We probably all know the story. It may be apocryphal, but it sets our scene, and there are many more examples. A mother sees her child run over by a car. Driven by her love, and her visceral drive to protect the infant, she rushes to the scene and, exercising strength far beyond what we should expect, seizes the bumper and lifts the vehicle off her child, thereby saving her from death or permanent disability. It's a high bar to reach, but it symbolises the power of action driven by concern for the other. Graphically, it demonstrates the extra dimension that the 'kindness' inherent in kinship and the willingness and ability to apply oneself to the service of the other can bring to a situation of risk and vulnerability. It says that kindness moves mountains.

But look at it another way. The mother made no risk assessment. She had no training in handling and lifting. She ignored the evidence that a car was unliftable. She intervened in a way that encroached upon the responsibilities of other services – the police, the fire brigade, the ambulance service. She almost certainly left other things unattended to – perhaps another child in the kitchen with a boiling pan on the stove, perhaps another made late for school. She didn't record the incident to enable later evaluation. She gave herself a back injury requiring care over the years, culminating in absence from work and several expensive operations. She was over-involved. She was irresponsible and out of control. The story surely illustrates the need for systems, skills, evidence, evaluation and regulation, and the cost of ill-managed care.

How do we read this contradictory picture? Almost certainly, we all feel that the remarkable act was the right one, and we would hope to be so transformed by kindness if it was our own child. Again, almost certainly, we would hope that we were always ready to 'go the extra mile' for our friends, our neighbours, our patients, though the bond, the sense of import and responsibility, and the actions we are ready and able to take, may be less as we consider these groups. As our roles and responsibilities become more sophisticated or professional, we become aware of the need to ration our commitment, to distance and preserve ourselves sufficiently so we can offer the most to the many. Accountable for working with the many, however much we pride ourselves on attending to the individual, we naturally look to evidence, to trends, to statistically analysed choices to help us decide what to do. Working with the many, we are exposed to risk and anxiety day after day. We know we get tired, we know we might make mistakes. We know problems are complex, and require, in turn, the organisation of a similarly complex range of highly sophisticated, evidence-based professional skills and interventions. We know that skills and resources are limited and need organising for the best benefit. We *want* to share the responsibility, we *want* things to be managed.

At the heart of the issue is a real tension between the kind of thinking and feeling elicited by focusing on how to promote kind, person-centred care on the one hand, and by standardisation, regulation and performance management on the other. We need to understand this tension if we are to release the potential for improvement in effectiveness, efficiency and patient satisfaction. Reading our story above, most readers will be able to imagine the feelings of the mother if anyone were to interrupt her in full flight to require her to follow 'procedures' – and perhaps what would happen to her child should she delay. The example is, of course, emotive and extreme: but the predicament is there for every healthcare worker, who must work within the tension between being free to act as an individual in response to the needs of the patient and being accountable for following rules.

The second narrative has predominated in recent years: standardisation and target setting, regulation, performance management and systematis-ation of care, doing things efficiently, applying evidence, inspecting. Society has, to a large extent, placed its hopes for better healthcare in the realm of structural and regulatory reform. But insufficient attention has been given to thinking about how these processes influence the mindset and culture of organisations and their staff, and their consequent effect on the conditions for the promotion of effective and efficient kindness.

Free to serve the public

The American psychologist Barry Schwartz tells the following story:

When some psychologists interviewed hospital janitors to get a sense of what they thought their jobs were like, they encountered Mike, who told them about how he stopped mopping the floor because Mr. Jones was out of his bed getting a little exercise, trying to build up his strength, walking slowly up and down the hall. And Charlene told them about how she ignored her supervisor's admonition and didn't vacuum the visitors' lounge because there were some family members who were there all day, every day who, at this moment, happened to be taking a nap. And then there was Luke, who washed the floor in a comatose young man's room twice because the man's father, who had been keeping a vigil for six months, didn't see Luke do it the first time, and his father was angry.

Schwartz concludes:

behaviour like this … doesn't just make people feel a little better, it actually improves the quality of patient care and enables hospitals to run well. (Schwartz video presentation at http://www.ted.com/talks/barry_schwartz_on_our_loss_ of_wisdom.html)

None of the job descriptions for these people, and none of the specifications for their tasks, described such behaviour. Although the technical content for the hospital cleaners' job description no doubt listed tasks that would minimise the risk of hospital-acquired infections, of slips and falls, and so on, nowhere was there a reference, says Schwartz, to *people*. It is also clear that an inspection 'against specification' would have found shortcomings in 'performance' and, in at least Charlene's case, possible disciplinary action.

Cleaners may have a lot to teach us. There is a tale about Bill Clinton making a visit to NASA. He encountered a janitor in an anteroom and, being a sociable sort of President, asked him what he did. 'I help people get to the moon', replied the clearly very focused and motivated 'ancillary' worker. The janitor demonstrates clear focus on the 'primary task' of the enterprise, and knows that – and how – his work contributes. He sounds proud, and the sort of person who would clean rather thoroughly.

Direct acts of kindness so appreciated by patients and effective do not emerge either from unfocused goodwill or from the carrying out of prescribed 'kind' tasks: they emerge as a result of a state of ongoing openness to and empathy for people, attentiveness to what is happening and the readiness to respond with intelligent, kind action. They are less dramatic than the actions of the mother in our story, but driven by a similar form of kinship and connectedness. This is clearly also true for Schwartz's cleaners – whose actions, driven by empathy and generosity, were indirect and, indeed, would not even have been noticed by anyone looking at how people were interacting with the patient. Somehow, they are all keeping the person and their ill-being in mind, and retaining the capacity to act as persons themselves, while carrying out an officially delineated task. They see what *matters* to the patient and those around them and shape their actions accordingly. They also seem clear about how what they do might affect the overall task of the ward and are confident enough to act accordingly. However much Clinton's janitor friend had walked past 'vision statements' reminding everyone that they are there to get to the moon, *only* if he understands the links between his task and the team goal, *only* if he believes he is valued, *only* if he is treated in a way that accords with the team vision will he genuinely feel that his contribution is vital, and pay attention to the environment and his fellows accordingly.

In considering how to promote kindness we are talking, in essence, about four things:

- how to promote and sustain compassionate *bearing of the patient/other in mind*
- how to generate imaginative *understanding of the contribution a person's tasks* can make to others' well-being
- how to instil in people and support a confident *belief in their own value and freedom to act*
- how to ensure that they have the knowledge and repertoire *skilfully and compassionately to act* to fit the circumstances.

However important the framework of policy, regulation and performance management for health services, there are difficult truths to be faced about whether they are creating these conditions for kindness. These truths require response and management.

The industrialisation of medicine

Closely intertwined with the effects of commodification and market philosophy in healthcare is the influence of the 'industrialisation' of medicine. Steve Iliffe considers this trend (Iliffe, 2008). He likens the pattern of change taking place in medicine in the late 20th and early 21st century to the process that converted engineering as a profession from a craft discipline to an industrial one in the late 19th and early 20th century. Concentrating particularly on general practice, he writes:

Medicine is changing from a craft concerned with the uniqueness of each encounter with an ill person to a mass-manufacturing industry preoccupied with the throughput of the sick. (p. 3)

These changes are driven by the huge increase in complexity of medical care. It is useful to remember that the vast majority of therapeutic interventions and diagnostic technologies have been invented since the middle of the last century. Before this, medical professionals used their clinical acumen to make diagnoses but had few therapeutic interventions at their disposal, apart from some very basic medication and surgery. Having so much more on offer brings the need to manage resources and demand in a way that ensures an equitable and efficient service. This shifts the focus from caring for individuals and their families to improving the health of the whole population.

Iliffe's view of this situation is that we are part of a massive qualitative change in the delivery of health services, a change that has its own internal logic and dynamics. There is heated debate about things like targets and financial incentives, but a failure to recognise these as symptoms of change on a much larger scale. While Iliffe is well able to see the logic and some advantages of this change – and indeed concludes by appealing to GPs to engage and influence the process – he does worry that it could lead to a constricted, impersonal work style, with limited responsiveness to individuals:

The process of change is not a mere reorganisation, but a transformation of an activity from a loosely organised enterprise with a poorly defined remit and wide scope for individual initiative, interpretation and innovation, into a predictable and prescribed series of tasks in the management of the public's health. It is creating anxieties among professionals about power, autonomy, and patient-centredness as well as concern among citizens about the motivation of professionals. (p. 7)

Iliffe illustrates a central problem. If people need to be 'free to serve' if effective kindness is to be achieved, how can the dynamics of industrialisation – in danger of pulling the attention in quite the opposite direction – be minimised?

An example of industrialisation in healthcare

To illustrate some of the issues, the national scheme for improving access to psychological therapies (IAPT) may serve as an example. There is no doubt this was a creative, enlightened idea. It involved the transfer of money from the Department of Work and Pensions to the Department of Health in the hope that money could be recouped in savings from sickness and invalidity benefit – an admirable and unusual example of joined-up thinking between government departments. The clinical project involved intervening psychotherapeutically at an early stage in a depressive episode in the hope that this would prevent the sort of secondary problems (stigmatisation, loss of confidence and status, breakdown in relationships) that can feed into a vicious circle and result in severe cases being referred to secondary care as well as the fiscal burden of unemployment.

This is an example of what Iliffe refers to, using a term from industry, as *forward integration*: an attempt to improve the system by widening it to include and control earlier stages (another example is the reduced incidence of strokes through GPs' monitoring and treatment of high blood pressure). The IAPT scheme addressed problems at a 'macro' level (the effects on the economy) and problems at the level of mental healthcare (the recurrent complaints from service users about the paucity of talking therapies available on the NHS). The large number of patients who fit the criteria for anxiety and depression meant the scheme appeared well suited to *mass production techniques*, with large numbers of staff recruited and trained relatively cheaply, producing a *high-volume output* that would make it easy to evaluate significant change.

Iliffe describes how industrial approaches to ensure efficient working practice and manage the organisation of production processes are characterised by six activities (Iliffe, 2008, p. 41). They are listed below, together with discussions of these activities in relation to the IAPT project, where there have been real attempts to organise this process properly, but also clear evidence of inadequate *mimicry* rather than thorough application of good industrial practice.

1 *The central codification of knowledge.* The scheme has at its core a strong commitment to cognitive–behavioural therapy (CBT) and, though the original policy encouraged a broader 'central knowledge base', CBT has become almost synonymous with IAPT. This focus was driven by early optimism, based on research, that suggested CBT was effective in bringing about relatively rapid change, and that it offered a potentially cheap, easy-to-deliver approach. In fact, the evidence base for CBT having a greater beneficial and more lasting effect than other models of therapy is relatively weak (Cuijpers *et al*, 2010). This has been largely ignored in the interest of quality control, the evaluative regime requiring that the same product is being delivered in as uniform a manner as possible. The choice of CBT is interesting, as it is a very individualistic model of therapy, at odds in some ways with Layard's whole-system analysis of why the prevalence of unhappiness is growing in our society.

2 *The standardisation of tools.* There is a highly defined process for therapists to follow, right through from the first telephone contact with the patient. Evaluation of that process is extensive and makes use of a number of standardised rating scales. Many in psychotherapy take issue with the idea of 'manualised' therapies (where staff literally follow steps in a manual), arguing that they take the focus off the therapeutic relationship and the potential for a personalised response. Rating scales for measuring change during and after therapy are also controversial and tend to be skewed towards a particular model of therapy. There are also issues about validity – specifically, whether what is being measured gives a sense of real change, in terms not only of symptoms but also of overall functioning. Some things are easier to measure than others but this does not necessarily mean they are the most important.

3 *The subdivision of labour.* IAPT is dependent on training up a lot of new therapists in a narrow model very quickly, a pragmatic approach that has tried creatively to address a gap in service that has been neglected for a long time. There are obvious concerns about such a large and inexperienced workforce, trained in such a specific approach without the wider perspective that a broader training and experience would bring. There is very good evidence, from the literature on counselling and psychotherapy (see Chapter 3), that therapist characteristics, particularly experience, are more important in predicting outcome than the model of therapy used. Moreover, most research on the effectiveness of psychotherapy comes from academic centres using highly trained staff. One worry is the capacity of inexperienced people with narrow perspectives and rigid methods to recognise patients

with more complex problems who will require much more complex engagement, assessment and sophisticated care planning, including the management of many kinds of risk. More worryingly, specialist psychological therapy resources involving more experienced staff have often been cut at the same time as IAPT has been introduced. This leaves the service without the resources to work with the people requiring more complex care. This is an approach that is not untypical in the NHS. A gap in service or unmet need is identified, an initiative is set in place – an initiative that occurs in the context of severe financial challenges – with the result that other perfectly good services, much needed, and vital in the wider pathway, are closed.

4   *Machines replace human skills.* 'First level' IAPT services use online therapy rather than expensive counselling sessions. First assessments are done on the phone. While there is undoubted evidence that such approaches can help many people with relatively minor needs, some are concerned about the effects of this form of impersonal contact on people with more severe problems, and their feelings as they enter an impersonal, mechanical system, when it is human contact they need.

5   *Incentive payments.* There are no incentive payments for individual staff. The scheme itself, though, has had some prestige, and been widely presented as special (which in many ways it is). The teams have been, at least initially, engaged in what feels like a very special enterprise. But some would argue that the scheme is being both over-idealised and over-measured (to evaluate its worth, particularly in terms of return to work), with the potential undesirable consequence that therapists will be more focused on the time-consuming evaluations than the needs of the patients themselves. The focus on getting people back to work is also likely to distract from other needs of the patient.

6   *Faster work processes.* All IAPT interventions are short and time limited, to allow a larger number of people to get help. While this is appropriate for many people, there are few areas of the country where there are properly funded care pathways for patients to move on to if they need further therapy. There is also strong evidence that, for some patients, short-term psychological interventions cause more harm than good – for example, opening up intense and dangerous feelings without the time and psychological containment to work them through (National Institute for Health and Clinical Excellence, 2009).

The IAPT example illustrates both the strengths of the industrial approach and its potential pitfalls, especially if it is implemented inexpertly and without reference to the wider system. One of the problems is the way such schemes are rolled out across the country with little emphasis on local adaptation, despite huge variations in existing services. So, for example, the IAPT pilot schemes were carried out in areas where there was little or no psychological therapy available in primary care. Such projects were understandably popular and successful. But in another area, where there was already a well-established service, the introduction of IAPT meant wiping out a good existing service, built up painstakingly over years, and retraining extremely experienced therapists in very basic, manual-based CBT techniques. Staff felt devalued and reported that they spent excessive time at the computer screen filling in evaluations of a therapy they judged to be far more limited than their previous practice. Many GPs complained that they had lost the personal relationship with practice-based therapists.

Drivers for mediocrity

'Benchmarking' is another (industrially sourced) approach to systematising, ensuring equity and improving practice. The assumption, as in the IAPT example, is that one can compare in isolation specific parts of wider systems of care that vary from area to area, to support standardisation – in cost and process, in skills and 'tools'. As well as the dangers of undermining effective wider local systems highlighted above, there is clearly a high risk of 'benchmarking to mediocrity' – given the variable and relatively low levels of investment in some services nationally. The ambiguous process of standardisation, however, goes to the heart of practice with patients. Incentives to get all GPs to use the same depression rating scale, for example, will presumably improve the practice of those GPs not so interested or experienced in mental health issues. Others, though, are infuriated by the narrowness of the approach, feel that their accrued clinical wisdom is redundant and regret the lack of person centredness.

Rigid thinking, and the absence of genuine understanding of the system into which a new idea is to be introduced, has damaging effects on services and people. The inevitable need to industrialise healthcare, in itself, requires very careful handling to mitigate the risks of depersonalisation. But it is far worse when the industrialising process is idealised, misunderstood, and implemented in ways that would concern an expert industrialist or manufacturer.

If techno-centric industrial processes are allowed to create an impersonal, deskilled, rule-driven environment, staff are very likely to feel like tools and machines, and patients to feel objectified. The industrial roll-out of standardisation risks reducing the choice, and depersonalising the work, of the clinician, just as emphasis is being put on choice and personalisation for the patient. Such a process can undermine trust in NHS staff and services. The public begins to see a choice between impersonal public healthcare, explicitly systematised and governed by industrial measures, and the lure of the privileged customer transactions of private medicine. In fact, of course, private health services have their own clear vulnerability to unkindness, poor practice and abuse, mainly driven by the profit motive, but also by the inevitable colouring of the relationship when the patient is a paying customer. This may be as in dramatic examples such as the alleged

161

compromised practice of the doctors 'hired' by celebrities, the increase in unnecessary cosmetic and other surgery, or less vivid but no less important phenomena such as private surgical units operating without safe access to emergency care.

There is clearly the potential for industrialisation to undermine the clinician's autonomy and sense of freedom to attend to the patient, and to threaten a consequent breakdown in trust between them. Undertaken within a limited and fragmented understanding of the complexity of healthcare systems, and with insufficient flexibility, industrialisation can become blind and destructive. But one aspect of industry permeates throughout NHS culture – the view of work as a set of processes requiring regulation and performance management. Like industrialisation itself, regulation is inevitable and largely desirable. However, it is not a neutral process: how it is constructed and managed, how it influences the behaviour of the regulated, and the general culture of regulation all have influence. Essentially, this is a question of how staff are enabled to manage the balance between the demands of accountability and attentive response to the patient. The nature of regulation inevitably evokes feelings and behaviours. Unless these processes are understood, and the lessons applied both to the way regulation is constructed and managed and to how clinical staff are enabled to keep the patient in mind, the effects of regulation on a culture of kindness can be devastating.

The culture of suspicion

One factor integral to the quality of kindness is trust. How much we feel we are trusted, and how much we trust others, affects our capacity to trust ourselves and act compassionately. Social attitude surveys show that trust is on the decline, certainly in the UK – a so-called *crisis of trust*. Prominent British head teacher Anthony Seldon, for instance, in his book *Trust: How We Lost It And How To Get It Back*, describes the move from a presumption of trust to a presumption of mistrust (Seldon, 2009): distrust as default. He links this to the move from seeing ourselves as citizens to seeing ourselves as consumers, a move that forms a powerful theme in recent changes within the NHS.

Philosopher Onora O'Neill discussed *trust* in the 2002 BBC Reith Lectures. She found that despite lots of news stories about (sometimes genuinely) scandalous cases involving public servants, in fact there was surprisingly little systematic evidence of growing untrustworthiness. Nonetheless, the culture of insatiable accountability and regulation is promoted as the way to reduce untrustworthiness and to secure ever more perfect control of institutional and professional performance. But, O'Neill concluded, accountability has not in fact reduced attitudes of mistrust. Rather, it has reinforced a *culture of suspicion*:

We have misdiagnosed what ails British society and we are now busy prescribing copious draughts of the wrong medicine ... requiring those in the public sector and the professions to account in excessive and sometimes irrelevant detail to regulators and inspectors, auditors and examiners. (O'Neill, 2002, p. 16)

O'Neill points to the need to give up 'childish fantasies that we can have total guarantees of others' performances' and urges us 'to free professionals and their public services to serve the public' (p. 59).

Staff feel this societal mistrust and suspicion, both at a general level and in their encounter with the complex systems of control within which they work. This experience, and the need to allay suspicion, to fend off criticism, threatens constantly to undermine the conditions for 'freedom to serve'. Clinical leaders, managers and the boards of healthcare organisations need to develop strategies for 'buffering' this culture of suspicion, for creating optimistic, trusting milieux within which staff can work creatively. This does not mean abandoning accountability: it means working to minimise the toxic effects of the suspicion that goes with it.

Obscure accountability

Clearly, the many shortcomings inspection has revealed (and caused) do not inspire confidence, and reinforce the need for standards and accountability. But the problem may also lie in where accountability lies, and to whom. Onora O'Neill recognised the importance of this

But underlying the ostensible aim of accountability to the *public*, the real requirements are for accountability *to regulators, to departments of government, to funders, to legal standards*. The new forms of accountability impose forms of central control – quite often indeed a range of different and mutually inconsistent forms of central control. (O'Neill, 2002, p. 53, original emphasis)

Consider the following example of confused accountability described by a consultant psychiatrist and clinical director:

There is a new requirement that all out-patients as well as in-patients should have an ICD–10 diagnostic code entered into the data system from the first appointment onwards. The message from my managers is that there is no option on this one. Now this might seem a reasonable enough demand, and indeed for many medical specialties would pose no problem at all, but the issue of diagnosis in some areas of psychiatry is a tricky one. Colleagues who run the drug and alcohol service, for example, are reluctant to have to stick such sensitive information on computerised medical records (increasingly available for scrutiny by employers and insurance companies). Reasonably enough they have asked for reassurance that it is possible to have a diagnosis removed once it no longer applies, but have received no response.

In the personality disorder service, we have always been wary of labelling our patients with a diagnosis many see as stigmatising. The diagnosis is based on the presence of a collection of behavioural symptoms such as self-harm, rather vague relationship patterns such as fear of abandonment and inner feelings such as identity confusion. Many of our patients manage to develop better ways of coping and no longer fulfil the criteria by the time they are discharged. It is generally considered poor professional practice to label people below the age of 21 with such a diagnosis, as their personalities are still forming and who would want to be stuck with a diagnosis based on their behaviour as an adolescent? Even with patients where the diagnosis is appropriate, I would usually take my time to get to know the person, wanting to assure myself that the symptoms were enduring rather than a reaction to recent trauma and wanting to rule out other diagnoses. Forging a trusting relationship with our patients is all important and a clumsily imposed diagnosis could easily make it a non-starter.

So what to do? Stick to my ground, risk financial penalties and perhaps attract suspicion to the service? Swallow my professional judgement and, if challenged by an understandably angry patient, wipe my hands of the decision and blame 'the system'? Distract the patients from therapy and encourage them to protest? (Personal reflection – PC)

The rationale for the requirement includes greater accountability and transparency. Funders want to know more about what they are paying for and whether it is going to the right people so they can make decisions about future commissioning. There is nothing so wrong with that. But it is difficult to see how this will benefit the public. They have certainly not asked for the information or been consulted on the requirement, and are, we know, at the very least, extremely concerned about confidentiality. The example illustrates how central demands to specify and count can actually put pressure on the clinician to behave unprofessionally – to place accountability to regulators before responsibility to the patient. The incompatible requirement invites compromise and evasion.

The process (and detail) of specification and measurement, of definition of the task, is problematic not only in itself. The example shows how its mechanics 'outrank' professional judgement, and 'divide loyalties' for the worker between patient and funder, between public and government. The dilemma drives us further from personalised care for patients and makes real accountability more elusive. Further complicating the matter is that the source for and authority for the demand – the place where the issue could be properly debated – is impossible to find. This 'source' is actually a complex and inaccessible web of professional, policy, commissioning, contracting and information technology bodies and interests.

Regulation, then, occurs within a mistrustful culture. The demands of regulators can be at odds with patient care, and the system frequently makes it hard for staff to negotiate these problems. Regulation also involves competition – through league tables, outcome comparisons, performance rankings and so on. In organisations already infused with anxiety about competition within a market, this mix of forces can powerfully reinforce the pull towards perversion.

The dangers of standardisation and competitive regulation

The extreme cases tell an obvious story. There are performance-driven activities that kill, especially within the culture of mistrust within which they are working. The drive to cut costs while meeting targets for waiting times in accident and emergency departments was apparently translated in the Mid-Staffordshire Trust into actions that included delegating, albeit unofficially, complex triage responsibilities to unqualified reception staff. The trust reduced ward staffing catastrophically, despite staff protest. Many are likely to have died as a consequence, and many suffered indignities that verge on the barbaric (Francis, 2010).

There are other activities that increase risk, obscure and mislead. As O'Neill pointed out, the real enemy of trust is deception. Some hospitals reduced 'trolley waits' by such measures as redesignating the status of hitherto non-clinical areas so that they could be regarded (meaninglessly) as admissions. Some introduced 'hello nurses' – who did little more than greet the patient – to obscure the fact that people still waited for genuine assessment. Ambulances waited to bring patients into the emergency department to avoid them being recorded as waiting too long after arrival. In other places, people cheated and figures relating to targets were simply 'massaged'. Hospital managers deliberately misrepresented records to make their performance look better. This picture has been widespread:

More than 6,000 patients suffered when hospital managers deliberately massaged waiting list data to hide the fact that they were missing government targets for shorter queues. Some patients were forced to wait much longer than they should have done and Nigel Crisp, the chief executive of the NHS, has accepted that the health of some may have deteriorated. (House of Commons Public Accounts Committee, 2002)

Such stories demonstrate behaviour that damages the enterprise of improving – at times even delivering – healthcare. The stories involve the participation of many people. They are illustrations of the dangers of approaches driven by target or performance indicators, unmitigated by ethics, disconnected from the reality of patient need and experience. Some may well be frankly perverse, in the sense discussed earlier. Some show all the signs of high anxiety and panic, scarcely contained and leaking out into desperate unconsidered action. Some are just unreflective, unsubtle, unhelpful.

These examples are extreme and are probably not the norm – though not as rare as the numbers of such activities that have come to light. But they are an extreme on a spectrum: the dynamics they illustrate are present wherever governance, performance and quality management are less dramatically, but no less clumsily, (mis)handled.

Unintended consequences

There is evidence that, as well as supporting improvement, target- or indicator-driven activities can have, in themselves, a range of unhelpful unintended consequences. Researchers from the University of York and the University of St Andrews report a range of such consequences (Goddard *et al*, 2000). They have found consistent evidence of:

- *tunnel vision* – concentration on areas that are included in the performance indicator scheme, to the exclusion of other important areas
- *suboptimisation* – the pursuit of narrow local objectives by managers, at the expense of the objectives of the organisation as a whole
- *myopia* – concentration on short-term issues, to the exclusion of long-term criteria that may show up in performance measures only in many years' time
- *measure fixation* – focusing on what is measured rather than the outcomes intended
- *complacency* – a lack of motivation for improvement when comparative performance is deemed adequate
- *ossification* – referring to the organisational paralysis that can arise from an excessively rigid system of measurement
- *misrepresentation* – the deliberate manipulation of data, including 'creative' accounting and fraud, so that reported behaviour differs from actual behaviour.
- *gaming* – altering behaviour so as to obtain strategic advantage.

Steve Iliffe covers similar ground, describing the risks of a system where economic factors outweigh professional imperatives in shaping GPs' behaviour. He describes three main risks: poor performance in domains where performance is not measured; hitting the target but missing the point; and discrepancies in data recording (Iliffe, 2008, p. 112). Even Chris Ham, health policy academic and head of the King's Fund, and a proponent of performance targets, acknowledges the dangers of disempowering front-line staff, stifling innovation and overloading the organisations providing care to patients (Ham, 2009). To this list we might add cynicism, disengagement and low morale in staff, and anxiety and mistrust in patients.

Targets such as those for waiting times in the NHS, although they have clearly worked to make access to services across the country better, can lead to lack of flexibility in relation to those who require more and less urgent responses. The focus on waiting lists themselves can distort the delivery and the quality of other elements of the 'care pathway'. An example here would be the way in which the laudable attempt locally to guarantee access to endoscopy investigations within 14 days had the effect of requiring patients to travel in all directions to various healthcare settings, some of them far from home. We heard, for example, of an understandably anxious Asian man, with little English, living two minutes walk from a city hospital, having to negotiate his way on two buses and a train, and a very different, rural, culture, because of this inflexible standard.

The systems thinker John Seddon comprehensively savages the public sector target-driven 'system reform' approach in his book *Systems Thinking in the Public Sector* (Seddon, 2008). He is a proponent of a 'pure systems' approach, centring on constant attempts to understand and improve the process of delivering consumer value rather than on imposed performance standards. Seddon warns that the focus on standardisation means it pushes services ever towards failing to meet the inevitable variety of the circumstances and needs of the customer. This plants the seeds of longer-term failure while making short-term, small 'improvements' in performance. Seddon, echoing many of the York findings above, identifies the following problems:

- cheating
- placing the interests of the (political and regulatory) regime before those of the people who need the service
- a focus on transactions and activity – in terms of quantity, timing and cost – instead of focusing on understanding what is of value to the 'customer' and examining the effectiveness of how the organisation delivers it or fails to do so
- fragmentation of the way in which a service works to meet user need
- added cost, in that attention to fragmented activity misses paying attention to fundamental wasted or misdirected effort
- a command-and-control approach to management
- a culture that sees people as requiring rules, direction, even coercion, rather than being motivated and intelligent about their work, identifying and solving problems, and being flexible in the variety of ways they need to work to deliver what service users need
- diminished initiative and imagination, empty conformism and rote behaviour.

These are not the conditions likely to promote the perceptive, generous, autonomous and person-focused behaviour illustrated by Schwartz's cleaners.

An alternative approach would pass the responsibility and power of inspection into the hands of those delivering the service, and reduce the split between them and a scrutinising and regulatory management. Management would focus on intelligent intervention within the system to address problems and opportunities identified by, but beyond the control of, individual staff or functions. Seddon points to a culture where the commitment, intelligence and goodwill of front-line staff are recognised and fostered, and where attention and resources are constantly focused on how successful the service is in meeting user need and on solving problems. If there are to be measures, they should derive from the work towards offering value, not from a form of top-down engineering.

Such a culture is more likely to sustain and promote attentive, kind work than one which mistrusts and reduces the autonomy of staff, and which overwhelms them with excessive demands to count and measure activity for the sake of fragmented targets or standards. Such a culture does not over-specify a list of things that should be done – though it fosters the use of effective methods. This is not a model that sees the delivery of, say, a written care plan, an offer of choice, a review meeting or the giving of a personalised budget as evidence of quality and value. They may all be valuable in any one of many cases, but the emphasis is not on illustrating quality by counting such inputs, nor promoting value by focusing staff on delivering a list of them.

As O'Neill (2002) advises, intelligent accountability requires more attention to good governance and obligations to tell the truth. It is important to distinguish here between two extremes in the culture of governance. One, increasingly dominant, absorbs time, work, money and attention in the process of developing more and more policies and procedures – that *demonstrate how* (though not automatically *that*) the organisation will meet a dizzying range of external demands. The other creates the space for reflective critical attention to the work of delivering value to the patient – and enables front-line staff genuinely and directly to *regulate their own work*.

Good governance is possible only if institutions are allowed some margin for self-governance of a form appropriate to their particular task. There should certainly be a place for professionals and institutions to be called to account, but this must not be at the cost of their being free and encouraged to address the quality of their service directly.

A more facilitative model

One standardisation project that tried very hard to avoid some of the unintended consequences described above is the Quality Improvement Network of Therapeutic Communities (Haigh & Tucker, 2004). Importantly, this was a *collaborative partnership* between the Royal College of Psychiatrists' Research Unit (RCPRU) and the Association of Therapeutic Communities. More recently, the RCPRU has rolled out the approach with other partner organisations to include residential facilities for people with intellectual disabilities, care homes for elderly people and psychiatric intensive-care units. Two nurses involved in the project described their experience as follows:

The first year was really difficult. We'd had quality monitoring visits before, organised by the Trust and the Health Authority, but they tended to be a bit irritating with lots of questions that seemed irrelevant and sometimes the reports just showed how little they'd understood about therapeutic communities and the patients we work with. So signing up to be part of this new quality network seemed an awful lot of extra work and we were all a bit defensive and worried about explaining what we do to outsiders. Because everyone was anxious, it was very much left up to senior staff to present things. But if your therapeutic community is involved in the project, you also get to send two staff members and two service users (along with someone working for the Network) to visit another unit and that was really interesting because you get to see how others do things and realise there are some things we could improve but other things we do really well. In general, we find we always miss out the achievements and have a tendency to mark ourselves down. It's hard when you're working day-in, day-out, to see the progress.

Each year it comes round, we feel more confident and it sort of frees us up to think afresh about things. After the first year, we made the decision to involve everyone at every stage of the process – that's all the staff and all the members [patients]. It's nice to have the chance to welcome people and show them what we do and getting the feedback at the end of the day, usually leaves us in a real buzz! Despite the exhaustion! It's not that all the feedback is positive, but the criticism is usually about things we know we're not so good at and it often comes with helpful suggestions.

It's so useful to take time out to struggle with the big questions: Why do we do it like that? Who has authority to make decisions? What do we want to do different next year? What are we proud of? And to be honest, we probably wouldn't do that in the same way without a bit of a push! It's really helpful to have the members involved. It seems really important that we step back and look at what we do with the people we do it for. It also makes them [the patients] question things and often they come up with really useful suggestions. Sometimes it helps them get things in perspective, specially when they meet patients from other units and compare notes! And the visits to other units with them are a really good shared experience. We also send a few staff and patient reps to the annual Quality Network event in London which is a chance to talk about our experience and influence the process for the following year. (Sara Moore and Juanna York, Francis Dixon Lodge, Leicester, East Midlands, in personal communication)

While the process described here demanded a lot of staff time, the effort was clearly felt to be worthwhile and relevant. Some of the factors that define this particular project and contribute to it being a positive experience include the following:

- It is an organic process, sensitive to feedback from front-line staff and patients.
- Collaboration is reflected throughout the system.
- Extensive consultation occurs from the start of the project, with the original set of standards suggested by front-line staff and patients and a lengthy piloting stage.
- Standards reflect aspirations of staff and patients, who are encouraged to develop them further.
- Areas of excellence are encouraged and cascaded through the network.
- Standards are tailored to a particular patient group.
- The emphasis is on encouraging development of the particular service and learning from each other.

- All standards are written in accessible, jargon-free language.
- Ownership of the system is encouraged by the holding of regular stakeholder events and the involvement of staff and patients in visiting other units.

While approaches like this may be seen as costly in terms of staff time, the investment is dwarfed by what goes into funding regulatory and governance staff and the processes of 'top-down' governance.

Refining the approach

The coalition government that came to power in 2010 made much of the aim of reducing bureaucracy within the NHS, retaining only 'valuable' targets and moving to specifying and measuring 'outcomes' that embed quality and patient experience at the heart of regulation (Department of Health, 2010). There is much to commend in these intentions, but everything depends on whether such an approach is matched by a radical change in the culture. For a long time now, the mindset among regulators, commissioners and managers has been coloured by mistrust and the quest to control, expressed through invasive and fragmented specification, measurement and policing behaviour. That is not going to go away readily. Competition is likely to continue to preoccupy staff, add anxiety and, perhaps, to evoke perverse behaviours. The temptation to measure and drive disconnected processes will persist. The imbalance towards accountability and away from responsiveness will remain uncorrected.

If there is a genuine move to capture outcomes that have meaning for patients and clinicians, then space to change may appear. However, an enormous culture change is required to transform governance to facilitate reflective ownership of the quality and performance by the staff involved, driven by connection to the needs of patients. Attention should be given to understanding and addressing the workload pressure, the distraction from task and the emotions and attitudes evoked by an overwhelming regulatory agenda at the front line of service delivery. A parallel shift in resources will be required to facilitate such change.

But the problem is unlikely to go away. There will always be a range of discourses at play in health services – and in the approach to their improvement. Some are derived from industrial thinking, some from engineering, some from natural systems and some from complexity theory. Some are professional discourses and some simply political or personal styles and preferences. Many of these discourses are in potential conflict; many, if not mitigated through some form of humanising and value-based process, will skew and damage the art of caregiving. This danger is always there, and it would be unrealistic to expect the conflict between regulatory approaches and good practice entirely to disappear. Careful attention to the *balance* between regulation and autonomy is needed.

There is nothing inherently wrong, for example, with having to 'tick boxes'. In defence of checklists – often seen as an irritation and an interference – the surgeon, Atul Gawande points out that 'our stupendous know-how has outstripped our individual ability to deliver its benefits correctly' (Gawande, 2009). He emphasises the fallibility of human memory and attention and the difficulties of applying, consistently and correctly, the vast knowledge we have accrued. Apparently there are 700000 medical journal articles published each year. In the face of this much information and complexity, it is hard to argue against some attempt to distil what is important in the form of guidelines – and checklists if necessary. But Gawande's checklist message comes with a simple warning:

An inherent tension exists between brevity and effectiveness. Cut too much and you won't have enough checks to improve care. Leave too much in and the list becomes too long to use.

He also stresses the importance of teamwork (hand-overs should be a 'team huddle') and places the checklist clearly in this context: 'Just ticking boxes is not the ultimate goal here – embracing a culture of teamwork and discipline is'.

This simple discussion of an aspect of regulation captures some important principles:

- the fine balance between, on the one hand, steadying autonomy with some form of external control and, on the other, overwhelming the system with too many demands and too much information
- the importance of keeping the larger picture in perspective and keeping in mind how the fragment fits with the whole
- an understanding that any form of regulation will affect important relationships, positively or negatively
- the centrality of open, honest and disciplined teamwork that makes use of rather than accounts to regulation.

Perverse and destructive, or ineffective attitudes and behaviours clearly do not derive only, or even mainly, from standardisation, targets, inspection and regulation. Individuals, teams and organisations vary. Many people, after all, are not corrupted by having to measure performance, or by having to compete. Many can keep a reasonable eye open for the wood when they are being forced to count the trees. Many organisations have managed to reduce waiting lists and minimise the risk of distortion of the wider system. Thousands of patients are relieved and grateful that they have been able to receive interventions for painful and worrying conditions more speedily. Even staff who might not have prioritised waiting times have seen that the pressure to reduce waiting can have benefits, especially when the initiative is part of a wider focus on improving patient care. There is evidence of other well-set targets working: the incentives for GPs to actively monitor and treat blood pressure, for example, seems to be reducing the incidence of strokes (Iliffe, 2008, pp. 114–115). These successes should not be minimised;

however, we need to check that the focus on them has not undermined other aspects of care. They suggest that a balance can be found.

Finding the balance

Like any large organisation, the NHS is full of people on an ideological quest for the perfect regulatory system and others who think there is no point in doing anything until regulation goes away. But the plethora of (often incompatible) performance management paradigms is unlikely to fall away completely any time soon. The challenge is to find ways to promote the intelligent kindness required *both* to mitigate the potential for damage in these methods *and* to improve patient experience, efficiency and effectiveness. This challenge involves recognising the uncomfortable reality that the industrialisation of healthcare, the development of a competitive market and regulatory processes, however expertly or ineptly applied, will *always* tend to draw healthcare staff's attention away from here-and-now possibilities for effective kindness. Better to find ways of sustaining and promoting that kindness than to wait for some whole-system, coherent and faultlessly benign 'reform paradigm'. Better to develop ways of helping staff manage the tension than to wait for it to go away.

The individual healthcare worker is inevitably pulled between responding and attending to specific, here-and-now need or difficulty and paying attention to standardisation and regulation. On the one hand, staff must recognise the personhood, vulnerability and ill-being of the unique patient, and the anxieties and resonances evoked for them as people in their roles. On the other, workers must bear in mind, attend to and serve the needs of the regulation regime. At the same time, staff need to cope with the anxieties and emotions evoked by both the caring task and the way in which regulation is carried out.

To manage that tension as people, staff require the self-awareness and support to recognise and process these feelings. They need to be aware of the risks of being pulled by their own anxieties, or by insensitive, excessive and even persecutory regulation, away from the therapeutic alliance with the patient and towards increasingly dysfunctional states of mind and behaviour.

There are many examples of this pull leading to perverse, even brutal, treatment of each other and the patient. Fig. 11.1 attempts to present this picture graphically.

In the circumstances illustrated in Fig. 11.1, the individual brings herself, and her motives, anxieties and personality into a role, in a team, in an organisation. Roles, teams and organisations, as well as having explicit tasks and purposes, are containers for, and often a theatre for, the expression of the fundamental anxieties inherent in the task. In the illustration, the realm of regulation and its technologies brings its own agenda and anxieties that pull the individual away from attention to the patient and into, at best, distraction and disempowerment, and, at worst, frank brutality.

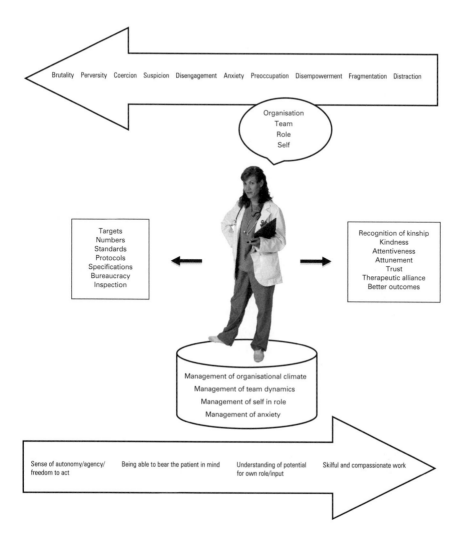

Fig. 11.1 The healthcare worker's divided attention.

It should be noted that the figure in the centre of the illustration could be a cleaner, a healthcare worker or a chief executive. A culture in which the achievement of standards and targets is primary will get inside all staff in an organisation and affect their values and behaviour, particularly if it is associated with mistrustful or coercive management behaviour, fragmentation of work and accountability, and general anxiety. Differing circumstances, differing personalities and differing roles will affect the level of tension, and the risk of the pull away from intelligent kindness towards

173

disengagement, perversity and abuse. Recognition of this dilemma is vital if intelligent ways of working to minimise the pull away from the patient are to be found.

References

Cuijpers, P., Smit, F., Bohlmeijer, E., *et al* (2010) Efficacy of cognitive–behavioural therapy and other psychological treatments for adult depression: meta-analytic study of publication bias. *British Journal of Psychiatry*, **196**, 173–178.

Department of Health (2010) *Liberating the NHS: Transparency in Outcomes – A Framework for the NHS*. Department of Health.

Francis, R. (2010) *The Independent Inquiry into Care Provided by Mid-Staffordshire NHS Foundation Trust, January 2005–March 2009*. HMSO.

Gawande, A. (2009) *The Checklist Manifesto: How to Get Things Right*. Profile Books. See also review by J. Quinn (2010) *BMJ*, **340**, c514.

Goddard, M., Mannion, R. & Smith, P. C. (2000) Enhancing performance in healthcare: a theoretical perspective on agency and the role of information. *Health Economics*, **9**, 95–107.

Haigh, R. & Tucker, S. (2004) Democratic development of standards: the communities of communities – a quality network of therapeutic communities. *Psychiatric Quarterly*, **75**, 263–277.

Ham, C. (2009) Lessons from the past decade for future health reforms. *BMJ*, **339**, b4372.

House of Commons Public Accounts Committee (2002) *Inappropriate Adjustments to NHS Waiting Lists. 46th Report 2001–2002*. HMSO.

Iliffe, S. (2008) *From General Practice to Primary Care: The Industrialization of Family Medicine*. Oxford University Press.

National Institute for Health and Clinical Excellence (2009) *Borderline Personality Disorder*. British Psychological Society and the Royal College of Psychiatrists Quick Reference Guide 78. NICE.

O'Neill, O. (2002) *A Question of Trust. The BBC Reith Lectures*. Cambridge University Press.

Philips, A. & Taylor, B. (2009) *On Kindness*. Penguin.

Seddon, J. (2008) *Systems Thinking in the Public Sector*. Triarchy Press.

Seldon, A. (2009) *Trust: How We Lost It And How To Get It Back*. Biteback Publishing.

CHAPTER 12

Intelligent kindness

The notion that ethics, altruism and fellow-feeling are scarce resources, whose supply is fixed once and for all and depleted with use, this idea seems to me outlandish – outlandish but deeply influential. My aim in these lectures has been to call this idea into question. I've tried to suggest that the virtues of democratic life – community, solidarity, trust, civic friendship – these virtues are not like commodities that are depleted with use. They are rather like muscles that develop and grow stronger with exercise. (Michael Sandel, 2009)

A change of mind

To apply the lessons from this exploration of the place of kinship and kindness in healthcare will require a radical change of direction. This change will need courage and imagination. It will need framing within a thorough application of *intelligent kindness*, an attitude and a philosophy that:

- unsentimentally values kinship and kindness, understanding their creative, motivating power
- recognises their effectiveness in driving quality, effectiveness and efficiency, as outlined in the 'virtuous circle' explored in Chapter 3
- understands what inhibits or liberates kindness at an individual, team, organisational or inter-agency level
- learns from and applies the body of knowledge on how to address these dynamics, valuing such work alongside other necessary approaches to delivering healthcare
- understands and mitigates the inevitable inhibiting effects of such processes as industrialisation, performance management, regulation and competition
- holds fast to the principle of enabling and protecting the 'freedom to serve the public' necessary for attentive, responsive and effective kindness, making, protecting and enabling this freedom the priority.

Without underestimating the difficulty involved, this reorientation is of such importance for the improvement and well-being of the NHS that it has to be made. Though the frankly horrifying excesses revealed in Mid-Staffordshire are extreme, the dynamics that produced them are *everywhere* in the NHS, and there is the risk that they could tip into such outcomes at any time, anywhere. These dynamics are at work in society at large, in government, the civil service and inside NHS organisations. Some of them are inevitable, and require recognition and management as the potentially dangerous forces they are. In the case of others, there is a choice.

Many of the examples used here to explore and illustrate the dynamics relating to the application of kindness have been negative. Abuse, scandal and processes working against good practice thread through the argument. The reality, of course, is that, every day, millions of people are being effectively and sensitively cared for by the NHS. However, this work is vulnerable, is becoming increasingly difficult to do, and could be far more effectively encouraged and supported.

At the centre of work to change the culture is the need to restore the emotional connection and investment that lie at the heart of the NHS. The government may choose to ask for more or less tax from the people, but the ethical, social and individual value of investing it in the NHS requires unembarrassed assertion. British society needs to reconnect with what a national health service means as a fundamental part of social capital, how it contributes to the good society, and how it embodies and sustains connectedness, equality and generosity. The idea that all of us suffer if any of our kin are neglected, and its mirror – that all of us are bettered by caring for our kin – needs unambiguous assertion. That it is a difficult, hazardous, uncertain and wonderful project – as a whole, and in every individual act of healing and kindness – needs to be made clear. These values and ideas require assertion across society, in schools, in public debate and in political manifestos.

A cynical, tax-averse, and to some extent state-averse, culture, with its frequent vilification of 'public sector workers' because they 'live off us all' and fail to eradicate some of the unavoidable horrors of the modern human world needs to be challenged. Healthcare staff work on our behalf, they express our willingness to care for each other, they wrestle with the never-ending complexity of our physical and mental health for us, and they face the difficulty of doing these things when ordinary people cannot or will not. They are human, and fail sometimes – especially when they are working with the most mysterious and frightening aspects of being human. Sometimes, they behave badly. How we treat them – whether through the policies we put in place to direct their work, the resources we allocate or the ways we regulate and manage them – makes an enormous difference to how well they work, for better or for very much worse. How we treat them is at least as influential on whether they are efficient or effective, sloppy or brutal, as the sort of people they are. The false and dangerous split between efficiency and effectiveness, on the one hand, and attentiveness and kindness, on the other, must be confronted.

Making this change also involves acknowledging that the current culture unquestioningly plays out hyper-anxious, mistrustful and often grudging feelings and attitudes. These attitudes are an understandable aspect of the public's connection with the NHS. They are based on a fundamental anxiety about investing collectively in each other and facing the levels of need involved. It is important to recognise that such attitudes are most prevalent where there is deep public anxiety and ambivalence about the condition or patient group involved, with associated wishes to deny or eradicate the uncomfortable nature of their needs. These feelings are the worst possible drivers for a successful health service. Pride, support and trust would serve better. Restoring such a foundation will involve positive assertion of the meaning and value of kinship as it is expressed through the NHS, of its ambitiousness, the sheer scale of its labour, and of its fundamental success.

Anxious ambivalence is most destructive when it is allowed to undermine the ability of organisations and their staff to feel and act upon a sense of responsibility and autonomy for what they are doing. The modern public sector organisation is rightly tied into accountability to society. But the more what it is doing is dictated and specified, inspected and measured from outside, the less any sense of a *capable community, focused on a common enterprise* can be sustained. The more the power is felt to be outside the organisation, the less it is owned and brought to bear on risk and creativity inside. Moreover, this externally based power, and the inherent anxieties behind it, affect the structures and behaviours inside the organisation, fragment the healthcare community, and blur the focus on collaboration. Collective attention to patient care inevitably suffers.

Regulating regulation

We must recognise that the culture and industry of regulation, management and governance requires rethinking. It is not a question of removing accountability, nor of abandoning the drive to improve services and achieve efficiency. But the current system, whatever its virtues in terms of identifying bad practice or achievement of fragmented targets, is not very successful at either *preventing* that bad practice or creating a culture of creativity and improvement. The answer is not simply to strengthen the current approach but to question its very philosophy.

The whole regulatory and management system should be seen to succeed or fail inasmuch as it helps front-line healthcare staff to work together effectively and kindly, focused on, and guided by, attentive connection with patients. Such a focus involves turning the current culture on its head. It is to envisage policy, finances and all aspects of governance as elements of an intelligently designed *medium* that will nourish engaged, effective kindness, instead of a crude *machine* for driving change from the top down, or from outside inwards. Currently staff are accountable to managers, who are accountable to various kinds of regulators, who are, in turn, accountable to government. Inside the organisation, complicated accountabilities are played out between managers, between departments and between professions. This is to some extent inevitable, but, at present, these dynamics are intrusive, over-complicated and distracting. Internal relationships, and relationships with the world outside, are too much coloured by anxiety and the drive to control, leading to organisational cultures of suspicion, coercion and competition. All too often, staff appear to be seen as untrustworthy tools with which to create organisational success, tools that need constant re-sharpening, re-organising and, to mix the metaphor a little, blaming, by the bad workmen who employ them.

It is entirely proper that society is concerned about the quality, effective-ness and value for money of health services, and that healthcare organisations put in place forms of assurance. However, unless a better balance is achieved between monitoring and promoting autonomy in these organisations on the public's behalf, the risk of poor-quality care will continue, and increase. Such a balance involves coping with an emotional challenge: how much does society express its fear and mistrust, or its hope and encouragement, in the way it monitors and regulates healthcare? The problem is that the more bad practice is identified, the more the first feelings are aroused, with their related 'technologies'. This is understandable, but not the way to avoid problems. Perhaps the biggest challenge in true risk management is to evaluate the risk involved in how we manage risk itself.

No amount of rhetoric about putting the patient at the centre of people's thinking will make a difference unless the culture in which staff actually meet the patients puts that clinical encounter first. Failing to do that is the most serious risk society and healthcare organisations face. This reality needs to be expressed in the values espoused by healthcare policy and organisations. It needs to drive the way resources, systems and people are managed and the overall way a healthcare organisation goes about its business.

Anxious, obsessional and fragmented regulation, combined with mis-trustful and instrumental attitudes to healthcare and its staff, create a toxic environment. This environment can, in turn, combine with staff anxiety and stress to generate a persecutory and overwhelming culture and workload that fatally undermines staff morale, disempowers them and further distracts them from patients. Can we envisage reversing the direction of this system? What if the whole system was directed towards accountability to the patient? This would mean, at the very least, reframing the accountability of the public, government, regulators and managers in terms of *duties to their front-line staff*, to enable them, in turn, to account to patients.

A minority of NHS staff may be lazy, stupid, careless or even brutal. There is no reason to believe that they are very much different from the rest of the population in this respect, although there are probably fewer outright psychopaths than in some other enterprises. If the public is worried about their work, what is important is to create a culture that makes it less likely that staff will behave that way, or more likely that people will recognise it when it happens. There is plenty of evidence of the effects of a poorly industrialised and target-driven culture, from inefficiency through to the perversions of neglect and abuse, to suggest current approaches are part of the problem. If people are willing to listen. The reports on Mid-Staffordshire, Maidstone and Tunbridge Wells and so on suggest explicitly that such a culture, as its labyrinthine wheels of clinical governance rattle on, has been a major factor in killing people.

The process of creating a culture that will nourish compassionate healthcare begins with daring to turn the focus from chasing poor practice and controlling people to supporting and enabling staff to do what they would in most cases want to do well. The shift means recognising the emotional work involved in connecting with and treating patients and ensuring that what is happening can be acknowledged and processed at all levels. It also involves explicitly and vigorously valuing attentive kindness. Kindness makes a difference at every level and can promote the virtuous circle outlined in Chapter 3. Our brains are programmed to respond to kindness and people are more likely to be kind and compassionate when they feel safe and cared for themselves. Importantly, too much threat in the system will fatally undermine the capacity for kindness. A compassionate healthcare culture depends on having the courage to trust the goodwill and skills of the majority, and the imagination to understand what they need to help them do their jobs well. Imagination is also required to understand the likely effects on staff and patients of *any* way of regulating and managing.

A mature approach to industrialisation

The change of focus required also involves restraining the current enthusiasm for uncritical application to healthcare of a technical, industrially inspired mindset. It means daring to consider the work as a *psychosocial enterprise*, involving human relationship, emotion and the capacity to think about and care for others. There are undoubted benefits from looking at processes and efficiency. But unless we hold the focus on what helps healthcare staff use their own personal and collective resources to face, make sense of and respond to patient experience and need, such an approach is bound to let us down.

A good start would be to understand when the industrial or business paradigm that will help is that of *production systems*, and when it is that of *creative industry*. The first requires a very different approach to the second. A film or theatre company, a newspaper, or the innovation department of a software firm are all businesses, aiming to grow and succeed. But successful ones have learned to put the highest value on the imagination, creativity and, critically, individuality of their staff. They have become expert in supporting and nourishing these qualities. Though many aspects of healthcare can be improved by applying a production system model, the vast majority of NHS work would benefit more from learning from creative industry. The NHS, because it aims to treat the whole nation, must, of course, consider what it does that is like mass production, and needs the best of such thinking to help with these things. But every minute, every day, before they reach for technology, medication or scalpel, human staff are trying to connect with, understand, calm and care for anxious human patients. Relationships are not units of production. If any industrial paradigm is required, then it should probably be drawn from industries that aim to deploy aware, autonomous and resourceful human creativity, not production-line workers.

Can we balance the traditional industrial view with another? Can we consider what will help staff with their *emotional labour* and support them in remaining *alive to* the moment-to-moment encounter with the people who are their patients? Can we support their central effort: that of managing themselves, their relationships and resources, and putting themselves at the service of the patient, attentively, sympathetically and effectively? Can we trust that they are better able to do things well and efficiently if we 'regulate' them in this way?

Kindness and efficiency

The act of courage required to reinstate intelligent kindness does not mean giving up ideas of efficiency. Staff inspired by attentive kindness will be more efficient than distracted, persecuted and depressed staff. When asked what will meet patient need better, they will tend to know, because they are genuinely in touch with and understand that need. Taking this stance does not mean sacrificing 'innovation' either. Staff attuned to patient experience and the effectiveness of care will be more open to intelligent, patient-centred reflection and learning, and genuinely committed to improvement, rather than mechanical implementation of prescribed models. Such people will be able to employ 'improvement technologies' more intelligently and to more effect.

Even if it were advisable to do away with them, which is questionable, targets and standards, or something like them, would undoubtedly still require attention. But the evidence is there to be learned from, and if the thesis of this book is accepted, there will be many fewer of them, and the regulatory framework will be much simplified and reduced. Money will need managing, and accountability for performance and quality will be required, but the way in which these aspects of good governance are presented to staff, and integrated into a medium in which to 'grow' intelligent kindness, will be crucial. A shift is required from bureaucrats, managers and questionably representative patient groups telling staff what to do, towards a genuine partnership of staff and patients educating and making demands on those managers, commissioners and bureaucrats.

Staff and patients need to trust the information they are given – about available resources, about the choices faced by commissioners and provider organisations. They need the opportunity to think about how to manage these things and develop standards and ways of evaluating practice. They need to be able to trust that managers will listen and respond supportively to messages, ideas and problems surfacing at the front line of healthcare.

Critically, they need to be sure that the public, politicians, commissioners and managers restrain the fatuous and uncritical (and currently widespread) assumption that there can *always* be 'more for less'. Staff, if properly supported by responsive leadership, will happily consider ways of improving services or making them more efficient. But the ideal way of stopping them doing this is to insult their intelligence by asserting that reducing resources and increasing activity and quality is *always* possible.

Of particular importance here is to challenge not the idea of increased efficiency, but the lazy, blanket expectation that *all* parts of the system can and should be able to generate savings and increase activity. This assumption – or behaviour that seems to reflect it – is much more common than the number of people who would admit to it. Closely related to this nonsense is the comforting self-delusion that increased demand and efficiency do not cost people effort – 'work smarter, not harder' has some value as a guiding slogan, but not when it is used deliberately to avoid counting the real cost of service reductions, increased demand, stress or reduced time with patients. Intelligent analysis of genuine opportunities for efficiency, and honest recognition of the costs and benefits involved, is likely to recruit hearts and minds to the enterprise rather better.

Whatever the fringe benefits of the enormous investment in regulation and inspection, it appears unarguable that a major source of the efficiency the public more than ever require would be the radical reduction of such investment and its redirection into services. The majority of senior managers and clinicians we have spoken to attest to the fact that more of their time is spent in responding to regulation than to leading, supporting and developing their services. Remove some of the need to 'feed the beast' of inspection, and immediately time and resources are freed up to improve services. Reduce some of the fragmentation, anxiety and distraction caused by the industry of standards and the work to meet and measure them, and attention returns to the needs of patients.

Leadership

It is the responsibility of leaders, in management and clinical roles, to manage the tension between the effects of industrialisation, regulation and task-related stress, and the precarious work of caring kindly and effectively for patients. This task requires careful strategic work to create an environment where all business and bureaucratic systems are aligned to promote the delivery of attentive, compassionate and responsive care. This may mean occasionally having the courage to subordinate financial and performance pressures to the need to ensure the right conditions for care, but that is not inevitable.

To begin with, genuine acceptance that a healthcare organisation is a psychosocial, as well as a technical or business, entity is vital. It will help if leaders understand that the psychological climate and the dynamics of relationships require at least as much attention and skilled, hard work as business processes. There is a common tendency to relegate staff experience to the realm of 'engagement', 'briefing', 'satisfaction surveys' and the like, and to undervalue their reactions as convenient or inconvenient side-effects on the road to business success. It is important to resist this, with the clear understanding that creating the psychological conditions for compassionate healthcare is a vital task – and that it is everybody's responsibility.

Understanding of the tensions at play between attention to patients, business processes and organisational climate can help leaders understand how processes can enable rather than undermine care. Ensuring that people with responsibilities in these areas are required, and helped, to think together, and to consider the combined effects of their activities, is vital. Conflict is inevitable, whether between priorities, between colleagues or between clinical staff and managers. Properly respected and considered, it can offer the leader evidence of work at the psychosocial level that needs to be done. Unaddressed, it can sap away compassionate focus on the patient. The capacity for leaders to keep in mind their accountability to front-line staff and patients, and to remain open, attentive and sympathetically focused on what they are experiencing, is crucial.

In the end, how leaders behave, whatever role they play, will make the biggest difference. The more attentive they are to the emotional reality of caregiving, the more likely they are to apply their imagination to how to manage potentially dangerous tensions and dynamics. The more they demonstrate authentically that they value and understand the emotional labour involved in work with patients, the more their staff will help them find creative ways of achieving objectives. The more they are seen genuinely to prioritise intelligent kindness, the more staff will cooperate and make that real.

The culture and values of NHS leadership need scrutiny – from top to bottom. It is understandable that organisations value people who can 'get things done', but too often that translates into promoting people who will skate over the real cost and complexity of the work, and achieve short-term targets at the expense of staff morale and patient centredness. Such people frequently appear to be unable to contemplate the possibility of unintended or undesirable consequences, especially of their own actions. Although they are not always bullies – and would be chagrined to think that they might be – their ways of working are often perceived as being close to that. The impetus to work this way could be countered were leaders to manage the anxiety inherent in their roles, and support and challenge each other when it affects behaviour. They need to be able to resist the urge to minimise genuine complexity and to denigrate or turn a blind eye to staff who either raise problems or fail to meet impractical, even impossible, demands.

Managing such anxiety requires personal qualities, such as maturity. It requires recognition of the dangers unmanaged anxiety can introduce and a strong collective commitment to helping each other stay open to what is really happening in the service's relationship with patients. Leaders need to be emotionally capable of trusting staff, brave enough to put supporting front-line practice at the centre of their thoughts, and alive and attentive enough to notice where things are going wrong. They need to resist the temptation to rule by fear and procedure and instead promote and model openness, participation and collective creativity and problem-solving.

There are many anxious, ambitious and reactive managers and leaders, some of whom are simply ineffectual, some of whom place healthcare secondary to organisational and personal success, and some of whom attempt to drive their staff towards achieving targets in ways that often include silencing or bullying them. Some of this behaviour, inevitably, springs from personality, but much stems from a culture of competition, punitive responses, confused accountability and unrealistic expectations.

It is a strong and wise chief executive who recognises that a large part of the job is to manage their own anxiety, to restrain their tendency to pass it on to staff, and to model and manage this approach through their fellow senior managers. An effective leader understands what their staff's work involves and can listen well enough to identify the barriers that make it difficult to do. A mature leader can ask, rather than tell, staff how to achieve difficult targets. An intelligent and honest leader recognises that saying that something is so ('we are a people-centred organisation', for example) does not make it so – resources, attitudes and skilled behaviour do. It is a principled and brave leader who is honest enough to accept and defend the real limits to what staff can do within the resources they have. It is a sensible leader who resists the lure of the role of hero and charismatic ruler of an organisation and instead strives to be the convenor of its community, the guardian of its conscience and the servant of its purpose. To work in these ways requires integrity, courage and imagination.

Such a leadership role is hard. It is exhausting to account to a suspicious and ever-demanding outside world, to invest emotional, financial and human resources into doing so, and to manage the constant anxiety evoked by an often brutally competitive and unforgiving culture. Leaders, from the top to the front line, can be forgiven for feeling powerless, with so much defined for them – priorities set, and methods for achieving them prescribed. This predicament is unique to the public sector, at least in degree. No share-holder group, no competitor involved in a hostile takeover, has the right, or the exhausting battery of tools, to divert and preoccupy the leadership of a private sector organisation in this way. Contract management, with its associated pressures, is, of course, challenging to the private sector too, but intrudes far less into the detailed processes of the organisation.

It would be easier if leaders did not have to manage the anxiety involved in the current extremities of competition and permanent instability, and in the sheer weight of unbalanced, intrusive and bureaucratic regulation. However, even if that environment were to be eased, real benefit will ensue only if leaders are genuinely committed to, and understand the task of, 'leading for kindness'. They need to be both willing and able to see themselves as there to *help front-line staff help patients*, and to translate that into openness to the problems individual staff and care systems have in staying attentive to and responding with effective kindness to the patient. This is not just a matter of attitude and behaviour, or of fine words, like 'our staff are our greatest asset'. Leaders need the intelligence and skills to focus resources on doing something about problems and barriers, supporting staff, and helping them improve the service they offer.

Hierarchy itself requires attention. There is, in any system, a tendency for anxious front-line staff to abdicate and pass responsibility up the hierarchy, to where they feel the power and capacity to cope lie. This tendency is matched by its mirror image – leaders pass responsibility down without the support that front-line staff need to make decisions, changes, to take risks. The steeper and more tiered the hierarchy, the more an organisation becomes sluggish, unresponsive, paralysed. Leadership and front-line staff lose trust in each other. The increase in size of many trusts through mergers, and the supposed 'business rigour' of such processes as application for foundation trust status, have actually led to *more* tiers of hierarchy in many places, and this needs serious reflection.

Some NHS organisations talk about 'flattening the hierarchy', and occasionally act to do it. When it has happened, it has usually meant stripping out tiers of 'operational' management, or widening management remits. But no amount of such engineering will make much difference if the attitudes and behaviour of front-line staff and management continue to be shaped by hierarchical thinking and displacement of responsibility. What is required instead is a genuine culture of collaborative planning and problem-solving, fostering shared power and responsibility, peer exchange and mutual support. Building, supporting and leading strong and reflective teams, with an understanding of what makes them settings for compassionate care, should be a priority. There is plenty of evidence that people work better when they have a sense of belonging to a team that knows them, and that is ready to help them think and to support them in their actions. Equally important is to ensure that there are clearly mandated ways for teams and departments to reflect upon and address together the task of integrating their work effectively.

Finally, it is important that managers do what they have to do *well*. Poor financial strategy and budget planning, ineffective management of resources and people, and a failure to align the work of the organisation to promote high-quality services are all too common. Such failures frequently go unconfronted. Any modern organisation that has to freeze recruitment repeatedly and sporadically, or make unplanned cuts, or neglect the care of buildings, unless significant changes in its funding or costs have been enforced upon it, has patently failed in its management duty. If overspend is systemic (and has to be hidden by such unplanned means) because difficult decisions and the plans that depend on them are being fudged, then leadership responsibilities are being shirked. The challenge is to address these problems effectively, without drifting into brutal leadership behaviour to do this.

Professional kindness

Shortcomings in practice are not, however, simply caused by the regulatory regime and culture of leadership and management. Individual workers and professions need to reinstate attentive kindness as a central and valued professional quality and skill – and to restore kindness to its pre-eminent place in the 'duty of care'. They need to confront the dangers of defeatism, the way cynicism creeps in, hardens the heart towards patients and colleagues and silences imagination, critique and commitment.

Like their leaders, all healthcare staff need an understanding of the personal and group psychology of healthcare to help them undertake difficult work in complex and stressful environments. Vitally, from the very beginning of their careers, they need help to understand and take on the responsibility for autonomous action where patient need indicates it is required. Such a culture includes the recognition that porters, cleaners and reception staff – as well as having much to teach clinicians and managers – should themselves be helped to see their contribution to patient well-being.

The disturbing way in which highly trained and intelligent staff, the vast majority of whom are well meaning and skilled, have appeared impotent effectively to challenge perversions in practice requires serious consideration. It is clear from the reports into many of the recent NHS scandals that the management culture has set the frame for much of the staff's behaviour, and that such a culture, especially in the Mid-Staffordshire NHS Trust, was toxic in the extreme. Many staff did raise concerns, through a variety of reporting systems. However, the reported tendency of professional staff to disengage, to collude, or to split, in the face of obvious and serious abuses is frightening. Staff have professional committees, associations, trades unions and Royal Colleges. There is an 'outside world' – involving such bodies as strategic health authorities, regulators, MPs and local authority health scrutiny committees. It is understandably difficult for individual staff, who have been ignored, or victimised, after raising concerns, even formally 'whistleblowing', to take their stories beyond the boundaries of their trusts. But repeated reports suggest an absence of solidarity within and between professional groups in the face of obvious dangers and abuses in the care of patients, and equally obvious damage to staff members themselves. Somehow, the collective conscience we might expect appears to have been suspended. Bearing witness, asserting the duty of care, seems to have been subordinated, or abandoned in many cases.

An aspect of this silencing of conscience appears to be resignation, even a cynical *expectation* that things will be done badly, with the consequence that clinical staff, even very senior people, have simply disengaged, individually and in groups. The constant change, reorganisation and disturbance of working relationships has also tended to undermine collective conscience and the willingness to act upon it. As well as inuring people to disruption and its costs, constant reorganisation can breed 'myths of progress' – for example, that what people are experiencing is temporary and things will get better. There are structural influences too. Governance forums at every level have often become venues for the ticking of boxes, agreeing procedures required by regulators, looking at numbers and targets. Even when they are nominally led by clinicians, they are frequently management forums, focused on achieving organisational agendas, rather than settings where the reality of patient experience can be properly examined. Such work would be helped by reconsidering the kind of regulation trusts must face, and by challenging the risk-averse culture, which so frequently shows itself to be earnestly filtering the bath water while the baby is left to drown.

There are many factors outlined in this book that go some way, not to excuse, but to explain the apparent powerlessness of clinical staff in toxic healthcare environments. The disturbing findings of the experiments reviewed in Chapter 5, highlighting the tendency to conform to the group, to behave according to role expectations and to collude with malignant authority, also shed light on what may be happening. Professional groups and organisations, like any other grouping, can degenerate into factional self-interest, power play and various displacement activities, all of which means their contribution to the assurance of compassionate care is undermined. Such behaviour is often partly driven by the attitudes of clinical staff themselves. Some of these attitudes can be reinforced by hierarchies within and between professions. Some are evoked by the genuine need to argue different professional corners in debates about service models, about workforce planning and about opportunities for cost savings. But why is it so much easier to challenge and argue points of *personal or uni-disciplinary* principle and nuance about plans and models, than to work together to challenge undisputable neglect?

In parallel to this question is one for politicians. Is it possible to move away from simplistic pieties about 'putting doctors and nurses in charge', to find ways of reinforcing their moral contribution and genuine creative influence in healthcare organisations? The idea that 'bureaucrats' can be done away with and clinical staff 'freed up' to lead and manage the current overwhelming business and bureaucratic agenda is breathtaking double-speak. Politicians have placed these near-overwhelming burdens on organisations, and, while they are there, they need managing. Clinicians have been trained to assess and treat people, sometimes to lead, and occasionally to manage. Sometimes, management is a welcome choice for a senior clinician, but generally clinical staff are of most value when they are being supported by effective managers to do what they are best at – delivering care. Rather than wasting their training and commitment in giving them bureaucratic responsibilities, the *voice and influence* of clinical staff need to be strengthened. This is not to encourage the proliferation of individual axe-grinding or heroism. Individuals raising concerns – or ideas – face high anxiety and vulnerability to being ignored, or even punished. Individuals may often represent fragmented, self-interested perspectives. What are required are ways of developing conscientious, compassionate collective thinking and action within and across disciplines. It remains to be seen whether the idea of GP consortia commissioning care can become a system where clinicians have a much strengthened, key role in the development of services, while at the same time keeping their main focus the attentive care of patients.

New forms of organisation?

Considering the damage done by the continuous organisational change that has characterised the NHS over the past decades, it is with real reluctance that we consider the organisational implications of our thinking about kinship and kindness. There are, though, some issues that cannot be ducked.

The first is that the purchaser–provider split has been expensive and wasteful. The impetus to develop ways of getting hold of cost, quality and change is not the problem. But what has happened has taken the focus further away from patients, widened the gulf between clinical and business expertise and created crushing bureaucracy. It has failed to manage the inappropriate dominance and cost of acute hospital care. The admixture of unproven – and ineffectual – ideologies relating to the power of market forces to drive down cost and improve quality has not helped. Into the task of developing models and specifying their implementation has been imported incompetent gaming, associated with attitudes that denigrate and oversimplify real difficulties and resource shortages. Creating a mixed economy of care *might* improve choice and innovation, but promoting the most primitive form of competitive environment, with associated disabling anxieties and defensive behaviours, has frequently had the opposite effect. Private sector providers have been idealised, and often given a far more lenient – and ultimately financially wasteful – ride as a result of the dogged and gullible application of the ideology of market forces. In a complex and vast enterprise, what expertise there is to address systemic problems and improve services has been diluted and fragmented, and its attention directed towards structures, processes and regulation that have little to do with improving patient care or real efficiency. The system has confused challenge with destabilisation. There is a strong argument – supported by key stakeholders such as the British Medical Association – for reconsidering this approach.

The French philosopher Paul Ricoeur talks about the loss of *ethical intention* in public life and the threat to kindness, care and generosity as the market culture becomes more dominant (see Simms, 2003). There is a strong argument that there are worrying perverse incentives operating within the NHS that undermine its ethical intention. These are known about on many levels but a blind eye is deliberately turned. As altruistic values become crowded out and eroded by market values, it becomes increasingly tempting to adopt instrumental attitudes to work and put personal needs before the common good in a way that is self-perpetuating and draws others in.

The need to change the nature of accountability, responsibility and leadership discussed above suggests some ways forward. Healthcare organisations must place accountability to the patient at their centre, and to front-line staff as their resource for meeting patient need close behind.

This imperative suggests the need to increase democracy and voice at a local level. The main political parties have various ideas about how to do this. Foundation trusts, with their local community membership and representative governors, and their *relative* autonomy, were a New Labour vehicle, along with the development of local authority overview and scrutiny committees. Healthcare social enterprises and cooperatives are promoted in the coalition government's Health and Social Care Bill. The Bill's focus on patient experience and quality of outcome are broadly positive moves, though the dangers of proliferating bureaucracy to measure them are ever present.

We believe, though, that the Bill's proposals very seriously threaten the expression of intelligent kindness in British healthcare – and we are far from alone. The behaviour of a government purporting to believe clinicians know best, while systematically ignoring their general discomfort and alarm in the face of the commissioning arrangements proposed under the Health and Social Care Bill 2011, has been depressing to witness. The government proposes that 80% of the NHS budget is managed by commissioning GP consortia. In parallel there will be almost immediate dismantling of an admittedly unrefined commissioning administration through primary care trusts. These proposals have been challenged by MPs, the British Medical Association, Royal Colleges, patients' associations, the NHS Confederation and many others. The arrangements involved open up the system to risks of geographical inconsistency, to private sector organisations playing out self-interest in providing commissioning administration to consortia, and to destructive competition – fragmenting local healthcare systems and threatening quality through price competition. The pace of change proposed is dangerous, raising the prospect of a severe amplification of many of the destructive processes discussed in this book.

GPs are very well placed to consider and make decisions about most healthcare problems, but the exclusion of senior clinicians from specialist areas from formal involvement and responsibility in the proposed system puts at risk the planning and delivery of aspects of care and treatment in which GPs are not, traditionally, well informed. The proposals endanger comprehensive, integrated care, especially for the most vulnerable and those with complex needs. The 'pause' in the legislative process announced in April 2011 may lead to some modification, but without radical changes the proposals remain dangerous. It would seem far better to strengthen the role of clinicians across all 'tiers' of healthcare and across professions as the shapers of the healthcare system, and to integrate commissioning with governance of quality and cost, than to risk creating a conflictual divide between primary care and the rest of the system. Step-by-step slimming down of the administrative infrastructure through such integration would seem far less dangerous (and costly) than what is proposed in the Bill.

There is a persuasive argument for transferring effective ownership of *all* NHS healthcare organisations to their staff, with executives and managers accountable to the membership. Such an approach would mean a much stronger influence for the majority staff – the clinicians. It would require an absolute commitment to there being arrangements to ensure that all professional voices are heard, and to the *clinical community* being ultimately responsible for standards and governance. In turn, arrangements for ensuring that such organisations were genuinely accountable for priorities, quality and performance to local communities – to their patients – would be required. The so-far limited effect of overview and scrutiny committees suggests they need rethinking. The marginalisation of patient voices to 'complaints and compliments', or to managed 'consultations', requires attention whatever happens.

New local arrangements might be introduced, involving *elected council members, formally empowered citizens and expert patients,* to hold health services to account for what they spend money on, how they deliver care, and its quality. Around this system might sit a *very much reduced and simplified* national regulatory and standards framework. Services would benefit enormously, in terms of their ability to concentrate resources and attention on the primary task of focusing on the patient, and in terms of staff morale, if all elements of the culture of market competition were removed. There are other ways of promoting innovation and efficiency, and, if variations in demand, or specific needs, suggest that it is best to purchase care from the third sector, that process can be done without exposing NHS organisations irresponsibly to 'market forces'. A mixed economy does not have to be competitive.

Exploring some of these ways forward would restore and sustain the connections involved in kinship – the shared responsibility and concern, the interdependency and the humanity. They might go some way to creating the 'medium' for the focus on and promotion of compassionate care rather better than current forms of governance and accountability. It is quite clear that were these ideas to be explored further, how they are implemented would be what would matter. There is an unfortunate tradition in the UK of crushing the intention and spirit of change in its implementation. Absolutely central to the success or failure of any such enterprise would be resisting the anxiety to control or to ensnare such new arrangements in an even more fragmented regulatory bureaucracy.

The key thing is to restore a balance. The emphasis on ideologically driven prodding, manipulation and incentivisation from the outside to provoke 'improvement' needs to be restrained. The balance – and the restraint – will come through putting the focus on learning from, and building outwards from, the central human activity of bringing intelligent kindness to the healing relationship. Promoting a culture and organising systems that liberate and nourish that work will set in motion a genuine and rich dynamic of reform. The challenge is to begin, in earnest, to apply our collective intelligence and solidarity to make this happen.

References

Sandel, M. (2009) The Reith Lectures 2009, Lecture 4: 'Politics of the common good', broadcast 30 June, BBC Radio 4.

Simms K. (2003) *Paul Ricoeur*. Critical Thinkers Series. Routledge.

Index

Compiled by Judith Reading

Locators for figures/diagrams appear in *italic*

Abu Ghraib prison 71–72, 75
abuse
    patients 51–52, 101
    staff 59
    see also bullying; Mid-Staffordshire NHS
        Trust
academic training for nursing 64
accountability
    intelligent 168, 170, 178, 188, 189
    local 189
    obscure 163–164
    to patients 178, 180
Achieving Age Equality in Health and Social Care
    (Carruthers and Ormondroyd) 110
acquisition, consumerist 12–13, 21, 139
age-differentiated attitudes 117
ageing 102
    see also elderly care
ageism 117
agency 22, 79
    see also freedom to serve
Agenda for Change contract 146
agonic/agonistic social functioning 126–128,
    134, 137
altruism 52
    crowding out 142–144, 187
    role expectations 72
    staff support groups 81
    training 63
ambivalence 77, 101
    and anxiety 102, 177
    to change 135
    to kindness 43, 46, 52
    to neediness 102–105
    politics of 29, 31
    see also fear/uncertainty; love/hate
America (USA) 19, 24, 29–30, 80–81
anger
    and change 132
    management 59–60
    mixed feelings 102

    with patient traits 61
    see also hatred; hostility
animal studies 126–128
anxiety 21, 45, 107
    about death 120
    and ambivalence 102, 177
    and change 131–134, 136, 137
    and choice 21
    defence mechanisms 74, 75, 77–78,
        107–108, 130, 132
    and healing 42
    and illness 53–55
    indigent 100
    managing 182, 183
    perversion, culture of 152
    staff 59, 109
    and teamwork 68, 79, 86
    and trust 38, 39–40, 43, 44
    see also fear/uncertainty
anxious attachment 40–41
armed services, kinship 10
arousal levels, primate studies 126, 127
artificial feeding 118–119
assumptions, unconscious 73
    see also unconscious motivations
asylum seekers 102–104, 145
attachment behaviour 40–41, *80*
attention, divided 172–174, *173*
attentiveness 37–38, 43, *44, 45*
    and change 136
    horrors of illness 54
    kinship, edges of 108
    primate studies 127
    training 63
attunement 43, 44, 45, 54, 89, 111
authenticity 16
authority
    and change 132
    primate studies 126–127
    staff relationships to 70–71
    see also hierarchies

autonomy *see* freedom to serve
awareness
    primate studies 127
    self 172

baboon studies 126
bad news, breaking 120
balanced approaches 170, 172–174, 178, 180, 189
Balint groups 80–81
basic assumptions 73
    see also unconscious motivations
behaviour
    defence mechanisms 56–57
    rationalisation 56
belonging, and teamwork 79
benchmarking 161
bereavement, and system change 134–135
big idea 19
Big Society 5, 27–28
biology of kindness 40–42
    see also evolution
Bion, Wilfred 73, 74
Blackwell, Dick 101–102
Blair, Tony 125
blame, culture of 58–59, 135
blind eye, turning 140–141
    see also denial
blood donation 143
BMJ (*British Medical Journal*) 129, 141, 144
bogus asylum seekers 102–104, 107
boundaries
    change 137
    empathy 57–58
    staff-patient 60
    team 85–86, 87
Bowling Alone (Putnam) 23–24
breachers, discharge targets 89–90
brutal leadership 183, 184
Buddhism 62
bullying, staff 66, 182, 183
bureaucracy 27, 97, 98, 170, 186, 189
burnout 52, 59, 61, 62

Canada 23
cardiopulmonary resuscitation (CPR) 116–117
care coordinators 96–97
care homes 149
    see also institutionalisation
care pathways 91–93, 98
caring clinicians 39
    see also patient-centered care
case discussion groups 80
CBT (cognitive–behavioural therapy) 159
central codification of knowledge 159
Centre for Policy in Ageing 110, 111
Chandler, Raymond 33

change, cultural 170, 175–177
change, system 125
    defence mechanisms 130, 131, 132
    disillusion 136–138
    future scenarios 186–187, 188
    for good 187–189
    and grief 134–135
    lessons from ethology 126–128
    organisational dynamic 135–136
    re-disorganisation 128–129
    system overload 132–134
    top-down 128, 129–130, 133
    and toxic environments 185
    unconscious motivations 131
Charity Commission 28
cheating 165, 167
checklists 171
chief executives, NHS trust 133
child care, commodification 143–144
chimpanzee studies 127, 131
choice 21, 22, 95–96, 161
chronic niceness 119
chronic stress 21–22
    see also stress
cleaning staff 155–156, 167
climate change 14
clinical community 189
clinical networks 94–95
clinician–patient relationships *see*
    therapeutic alliance
Clostridium difficile 133
clustering, social network analysis 25
CMT (compassionate mind training) 62–63
coalition government 2, 170
coercion 167
cognitive–behavioural therapy (CBT) 159
collaborative
    partnerships 168–170
    working 90–95
collectivism 17, 26, 137, 139
    see also common good; connectedness;
        interdependence; kinship
command-and-control approach 167
commitment 52
commodification
    child care 143–144
    National Health Service 142, 150, 152
    vocation 146–148
common good 16–17, 22
    see also collectivism; connectedness;
        interdependence; kinship
communication
    fragmented systems 84–85, 92
    and healing 42
    and patient satisfaction 33–34, 35, 43, *44*
    and teamwork 75, *80*, 86
community 1
    capable 177
    clinical 189
compassion 3–4
    case for 37

and change 136
and defence mechanisms 130
definitions 10
and healing 42, 43
less deserving patients 60
organisational changes for good 189
for staff 65
compassionate mind training (CMT) 62–63
compensatory healing 111
competencies 64
competition 12–13, 14, 29
and change 129
and leadership 183
in NHS 142, 148–151, 165, 189
primate studies 127
and stress 22
complacency 166
confidentiality 91, 164
conformity, social 69–70, 79
primate studies 127
role expectations 71–72
connectedness 1, 46
building 26
clinician–patient relationships 3
evolution 14
and kindness 10
see also collectivism; common good;
interdependence; kinship
consequences, unintended 166–168
consortia, GPs 187, 188
consumerism 12–13, 21, 139
containment 79, 80, 137
continuity, medical care 118
Cooper, Andrew 137
cooperation/fragmentation 13–14, 82, 139
care pathways 91–93, 98
clinical networks 94–95
collaborative working 90–95
fragmented systems 84–85
leadership 97–98
narrowing down primary task 86–88
organization changes for good 189
pulled in all directions 88–90
putting the patient at the centre 95–97
structural integration 90–91
team boundaries 85–86, 87
coping with change 136
see also defence mechanisms
corrupting forces 142
see also perversion, culture of
cortisol 72
cost–benefit analyses 144, 144–145
CPR (cardiopulmonary resuscitation) 116–117
creaming 150
creative industry 179
crisis of trust 162–163
crowding out: altruism 187
humanity 35–38
Cuba 19
cultural change 170, 175–177
culture

of kindness 167–168
workplace 125

DALYs (disability-adjusted life years) 144
Dartington, Tim 87, 137
Darwin, Charles 13
Dawkins, Richard 13
Death by Indifference (Mencap) 111
death
attitudes to 100, 120
defence mechanisms 115, 117, 119, 121–122
facing up to 119–120
hospital 116–117, 120
rates 19, 24, 79, 128
tax 110
see also end-of-life care
debt 22
deception 165
defence mechanisms 44, 56–57, 59
change 130, 131, 132
cooperation/fragmentation 86, 87
against death 115, 117, 119
against envy 23
against neediness 105
over-identification 57–58
primitive 74–75
repression 56, 72, 75
role modelling 65
splitting 76–78, 107–110, 112, 119
towards asylum seekers 104–105
see also denial
definitions, kindness/compassion 9–10
degree of separation, social network
analysis 25
Delamothe, Tony 141
democracy, local 188, 189
denial
death 115, 117, 121–122
in elderly care 110
indirect discrimination 112
kinship, edges of 113
perversion, culture of 140–141, 152
in teamwork 74, 75–76, 79
Department of Health 117, 120, 129, 148
dependency
fears 100
feelings about 101–102
management 60–61, 109
mature 137
needs 73
see also neediness
depersonalisation 61, 130
depression 21, 61, 72, 145, 161
deprivation see exclusion; inequality
diagnosis coding 163
disability-adjusted life years (DALYs) 144
see also intellectual disability
discrimination 101, 110–112
disengagement 185
disillusion, and change 136–138

disparaging kindness 12–13
displacement, feelings 56
dissatisfaction, and stress 21
    see also patient satisfaction
distance between people, social network
    analysis 25
distress, healthcare professionals 53–55
distributed leadership 133
divided attention 172–174, *173*
divided loyalty 132
division, social 22–23
do-not-attempt-resuscitation (DNAR)
    orders 116, 117
double speak 152
dual diagnosis 87
dumping 150
duty of care 63, 185
dying *see* death; mortality rates
dynamics, team 68–69, 74, 81–82
dysfunctional teams 78
    see also teamwork

Economist 115
economy of kindness 144–145
education/training 62–65, 80–81
efficiency
    cultures 112, 133, 148, 151
    and intelligent kindness 180–181
Ehrenreich, Barbara 41–42
elderly care 3, 102
    horrors of illness 53–55
    indirect discrimination 110–112
    institutionalisation 108
    market philosophy 145, 149
    patient satisfaction 34
    prohibition of flowers 36
electric shock experiment 70–71
emotion *see* feelings
empathy 37, 38, 39, 42
    boundaries of 57–58
    motor 64
    role expectations 72
    for self 62
end-of-life care 115
    death in hospital 116–117, 120
    facing up to death 119–120
    keeping life and death in mind 118–119
    kindness 120–122
    see also death
End of Life Care (National Audit Office) 121
End of Life Care Strategy (Department of
    Health) 117, 120
endorphins 41
engaging with ill-being 54, 55–56
enlightened kindness 17
Enlightenment 12
entitlement, patient 2
envy
    commodification of vocation 147–148
    defences 23

epidemiological transition 18
equality *see* inequality
Equity and Excellence: Liberating the NHS
    (Department of Health) 129, 148
errors, medical 11
escalating expectations 21
ethical intention 187
ethology 126–128
European Working Time Directive 94
evolution
    hunter-gatherer heritage 72–73
    kindness 13–14
exclusion 105–106
    see also inequality
expectations 185
    escalating 21
    staff role 71–72
experiment, punishment 70–71
The Experiment documentary 71

facilitative model 168–170
failure, fear of 59
Fair Society: Healthy Lives (Marmot) 19
Fast and Fair? (Parliamentary Ombudsman) 103
faster working processes 160
fear/uncertainty 23
    death 117, 119, 121–122
    failure 59
    of interdependence 30–31
    of kindness 14–16, 30–31
    managing 59
    of neediness 102–105
    of psychosis 100–101
    see also ambivalence; anxiety; love/hate
feeding, artificial 118–119
feelings
    disturbing 100–101, 102
    group dynamics 73
    helplessness 100
    regulation 168
    repression 72
    sublimation 56
    towards neediness 102–105, 106, 112
    see also ambivalence; anger; defence
        mechanisms; fear/uncertainty; hatred;
        hostility; love/hate
fixed price systems 150
flattening hierarchies 184
flexibility 166–167
flowers, prohibition 36
forward integration 158
fragmentation
    and leadership 132
    social 27
    systems 84–85, 87, 118, 149, 167
    see also cooperation/fragmentation
free market forces 13
freedom to serve 155–157
    accountability, obscure 163–164
    balanced approaches 170, 172–174

facilitative model 168–170
IAPT example 158–161
industrialisation of medicine 157–161
mediocrity drivers 161–162
promoting kindness 157
refining the approach 170–172
standardisation/competitive regulation
    dangers 165, 167, 172
suspicion, culture of 162–163
two ways of seeing 154–155
unintended consequences 166–168
friendship 23–24
    see also connectedness
fright–fight–flight response 72, 73
frustration, and good-enough parenting 62
funding, NHS 1–2, 4
future scenarios 186–187, 188

gaming 166, 187
GDP 20
gestures, kindness 37
going the extra mile 39
Gombe Stream Reserves 127
good death 117, 119
good-enough healthcare professionals 61–62
goodness of fit, organisational structures/
    demands of healthcare 130, 131
governance, culture of 168
GPs
    change, system 129
    consortia 187, 188
    disillusion 136
    incentives 147
    role in continuity of care 118
greed 139
grief, and change 134–135
Gross Domestic Product 20
group
    analytic approach 82
    dynamics 73
    pressures 69–70
    supervision 66
    see also teamwork
guilt 58–59, 61

Haigh, Rex 79–80, 80
Ham, Chris 166
Hamlet (Shakespeare) 56
happiness, and kindness/health 25
hatred
    management 59–60
    mixed feelings 102
    see also anger; hostility; love/hate
healers, wounded 52–53, 59
healing, and kindness 42–43
    see also outcomes, health
Health and Social Care Bill 3, 129, 149, 188
healthcare professionals
    anger/hatred 59–60
    defence mechanisms 56–57

education 62–65, 80–81
effect of horrors of illness 53–55, 55–56
good enough 61–62
support groups 80–81
healthcare reform 1, 29, 187, 188
healthy teamwork 79–80, 80
hedonic social functioning 126–128, 131, 150
helplessness feelings 100
hierarchies
    and change 132
    ethology 126
    flattening 184
    see also authority
high-volume output 158
holding 79, 80, 137
Holtz, Lou 33
Horizon (BBC documentary) 71
horizontal collaboration 94
horrors of illness 53–55
hospices 119
hospital deaths 116–117
hostility 66, 104, 107
    see also anger; hatred
humanitarianism 35–38, 189
    see also patient-centered care
hunter-gatherer heritage 72–73

IAPT (improving access to psychological
    therapies) 158–161
idealisation 108–110, 112, 130, 136
Iliffe, Steve 136, 140, 157–158, 166
ill-being
    asylum seekers 104
    engaging with 54, 55–56
illness, reality/horrors of 53–55
    see also mental illness
image, preoccupation with 21
    see also materialism
imagination 179
Immigration Removal Centre, Yarl's
    Wood 103–104
improving access to psychological therapies
    (IAPT) 158–161
incentives, financial 147, 160, 187
inclusion 105–106
incontinence 53, 92–93
indirect discrimination 110–112
individualism 12–13, 14, 29
    and change 137
    and kindness 15
    and kinship 29
individuation 62
industrial revolution 12
industrialisation of healthcare 4, 126, 136,
    142, 157–162
    mature approach 179–180
inequality 18–19, 28
    and health outcomes 20, 21–22, 26, 27
    and kinship 23
    see also politics of kindness

infant/s
  defence mechanisms 75
  mortality 19
infectious disease 18, 95–96
information systems, fragmented 84–85
initiative 167
  see also freedom to serve
injustice, social *see* inequality; politics of
kindness
inspection 155, 166, 170
Institute of Fiscal Studies 28
institutionalisation
  denial 76
  mental illness 105–106, 108
  social pressure 70
  trends towards 108
instrumental relations 139
integrated care pathways 91–93
integration, forward 158
intellectual disability
  feelings about 101–102, 104
  indirect discrimination 111–112
  institutionalisation 105–106
intelligence, primate studies 126–128
intelligent kindness 10
  cultural change 175–177
  and efficiency 180–181
  industrialisation, mature approach 179–180
  leadership 181–184
  organisational changes 187–189
  professional kindness 185–187
  regulating regulation 177–179
interdependence 27, 137, 189
  fear/mistrust of 30–31
  see also collectivism; common good;
    connectedness; kinship
internal working models 41
internalising the market 150–152
  see also market forces
involvement
  choice 95–96
  and healthy teamwork 79
isolation *see* loneliness

J curve 129
Japan 19

kindness 3–5, 33
  biological effects of 40–42
  and change 137
  and common good 16–17
  crowding out the human 35–37
  culture of 167–168
  definitions 9–10
  disparaging 12–13
  economy of 144–145
  in end-of-life care 120–122
  enlightened 17
  evolution 13–14
fear/uncertainty of 14–16
and happiness/health 25
and healing 42–43, *44, 45*
and individualism 15
and kinship 9–11, 13, 45
limits to 101
patient experience 33–35
perversion, culture of 152
primate studies 127
promoting 157
pull away from 51–52
seeing the person in the patient 37–38
and stress 43
therapeutic alliance 38–40
virtuous circles 43–46, *44, 45*
see also intelligent kindness
King's Fund 'Point of Care' programme 37,
  43, 64, 66
kinship 100–101
  collective 26
  and death 121
  fear/mistrust of 30–31
  and health outcomes 42–43, *44, 45*
  idealisation 108–110
  inclusion/exclusion 105–106
  indirect discrimination 110–112
  and individualism 29
  and inequality 23, 28
  and kindness 9–11, 13, 45
  mixed feelings 102–105
  NHS as expression of 3–4, 15–16
  overwhelming need 101–102
  promotion of 112–113
  and social capital 24
  and splitting 107–108
  see also collectivism; common good;
    connectedness; interdependence
knowing/not knowing 140–141
  see also denial
knowledge, central codification of 159
Kundera, Milan 51

Labour government 2, 27, 170
language, collective 17
leadership
  distributed 133
  fragmented 132
  and intelligent kindness 181–184
  mature approach 183
  organisational changes for good 188
  team 97–98
league tables 150
life expectancy 2, 19, 20
  see also mortality rates
limbo, asylum seekers 106
limits to kindness 101
Liverpool Care Pathway 120
local democracy 188, 189
loneliness 22, 60–61
Long, Susan 137, 139

love/hate, managing 51
  anger/hatred 59–60
  compassionate mind training 62–63
  dependency/loneliness 60–61
  engaging with ill-being 55–56
  good-enough healthcare professionals 61–62
  guilt/self-blame 58–59
  intrinsic horrors of illness 53–55
  over-identification 57–58
  psychological defence mechanisms 56–57
  pull away from kindness 51–52
  supervision/support 65–66
  teamwork 76–78
  training/education 63–65
  wounded healers 52–53, 59
  see also ambivalence; fear/uncertainty
loving kindness 11
loyalty 10
  divided 132
  social pressure 70

managed clinical networks (MCNs) 94–95
management
  anger/hatred 59–60
  anxiety 182, 183
  of change 134, 136
  chief executives 133
  command-and-control approach 167
  operational 132, 134
  performance 59, 142, 162
  uncertainty 59
Managing Vulnerability (Dartington) 87, 137
Margulis, Lynn 13
market mimicking governance 144–145
market philosophy 189
  contemporary 143, 145
  in NHS 126, 142–143, 148–152
Marmot review: *Fair Society: Healthy Lives* 19
mass production 158
massaging the figures 165
materialism 12–13, 21, 139
mature approach 182
  industrialisation 179–180
  leadership 183
MCNs (managed clinical networks) 94–95
measure fixation 155, 166, 170
mechanisation of labour 160
medicalisation of death 121
mediocrity drivers 161–162
meditation 62
Mencap: *Death by Indifference* 111
mental illness
  compassion for 60
  cooperation/fragmentation 87
  fear/uncertainty of 107, 100–101
  indirect discrimination 111
  institutionalisation 105–106
menu-based interventions 92
Menzies Lyth, I. 130, 131, 132
Michael report 111

Mid-Staffordshire NHS Trust vii
  and cultural change 175–176
  denial 76
  neglect/abuse of patients 51–52
  mortality rates 128
  perversion, culture of 141
  regulating regulation 179
  social pressure 70
  staff bullying 66
  standardisation/competitive regulation
    dangers 165
  and system change 133
  teamwork 73, 78
  toxic environments 185
mind training, compassionate (CMT) 62–63
mindfulness 62–63
mirror neurons 64
misrepresentation 166
mistakes, medical 11
mistrust *see* trust/mistrust
mixed economy 142, 148, 189
mixed feelings *see* ambivalence
morale, staff 44, 178
  Agenda for Change 146–147
  and change 136
  and healthy teamwork 79
  and kindness 46
  see also patient satisfaction
morality, role expectations 72
mortality rates 2, 19, 24, 79, 128
  see also death; end-of-life care; life expectancy
mother love vignette 154–155
motivation, health-care professionals 52–55
  see also unconscious motivations
mutuality, and change 137
  see also collectivism; common good;
    connectedness; cooperation/
    fragmentation; interdependence; kinship
myopia 166

narcissism 139
National Centre for Social Research
  (NCSR) 26, 27
National Confidential Enquiry into Patient
  Outcomes and Death (NCEPOD) 85,
  116, 117, 118, 120, 121
National Equality Panel (NEP) 26
National Health Service 1–6, 15–16
  chief executives 133
  contemporary 139
  market forces 142–143, 148–152
  need for cultural change 176
  perversion, culture of 148–50
  promotion of kindness 10
  reorganisation 125
NCEPOD (National Confidential Enquiry
  into Patient Outcomes and Death) 85,
  116, 117, 118, 120, 121
NCSR (National Centre for Social
  Research) 26, 27

neediness
  feelings towards 102–105, 106, 112
  overwhelming 101–102
  and teamwork 79
  see also dependency
negativity 102
  see also feelings
neglect/abuse of patients 51–52, 101
  see also Mid-Staffordshire NHS Trust
NEP (National Equality Panel) 26
networks, clinical 94–95
neurobiology of kindness 40–42
NHS *see* National Health Service
The NHS Plan 129
niceness, chronic 119
Nietzsche, F. 68
nursing staff
  academic training 64
  study 130, 131, 132

Obama, Barack 29, 30
objectification of patients 161
objective situation 130
objectivity, and kindness 145
obsessive–compulsive symptoms 72
OFSTED guidelines on child care 143–144
  see also inspection
omnipotence, health-care professionals
      121–122, 131
On Kindness (Phillips and Taylor) 12, 14
O'Neill, Onora 162–163
openness 39, 85
operational managers 132, 134
organisation/al
  changes for good 187–189
  dynamic 135–136
  goodness of fit 130, 131
  in the mind 125, 138
The Origin of Species (Darwin) 13
ossification 166
otherness 101, 105, 106
outcomes, health
  and inequality 18–22, 26, 27
  and kindness 25, 38, 42–43, *44, 45*
  and kinship *44, 45*
  measurement 155, 166, 170
  and social capital 23–25
over-identification, healthcare
professionals 57–58
overwhelming need 101–102
oxytocin 41

pain relief 34
palliative care 119, 120
panic attacks 72
The Paradox of Choice: Why More is Less
      (Schwartz) 21
paralysis, and choice 21
Parliamentary Ombudsman: *Fast and Fair?* 103

part-object relating 118
passivity, teamwork 79
pathways, care 91–93, 98
patient/s 5–6
  accountability to 178, 180
  distress, dealing with 54
  neglect/abuse 51–52, 101
  objectification 161
  undeserving 60, 100
patient-centered care 35–38, 95–97, 172,
      180, 182, 184, 187, 189
patient satisfaction 1, 4
  case for kindness 33–35
  and communication 43, *44*
  and kindness 16, 43, 46
performance
  management 59, 142, 162
  targets 165
personalisation 95
personality disorder 163–164
personhood, recognition 172
  see also patient-centered care
perspectives, two ways of seeing 154–155
The Perverse Organisation and Its Deadly Sins
      (Long) 139
perversion, culture of 164, 172, 174
  altruism, crowding out 142–144
  commodification of vocation 146–148
  corrupting forces 142
  incentives 187
  internalising the market 150–152
  kindness, economy of 144–145
  knowing/not knowing 140–141
  NHS market 148–150
  perverse dynamics 139–140
  standardisation/competitive regulation
      dangers 166
Phillips, Adam 12, 14
physician, heal thyself 53
Pickett, Kate 20, 30
placebo effect 42
'Point of Care' programme, King's Fund 37,
      43, 64, 66
polarisation 108, 110
  and change 135
  thinking 101
  see also splitting
politics
  ambivalence 29–31
  and change 129
  chronic stress 21–22
  coalition government 2, 170
  impact on NHS 1–3, 5
  implications 26–29
  and kindness 11, 18, 25
  local democracy 188, 189
  poverty and health 18–19, 26
  social capital and health 23–25
  social division 22–23
  see also inequality
positive regard 39, 42

positive thinking 41–42, 136
  see also idealisation
possessions, materialist 12–13, 21, 139
post-traumatic stress 103
poverty *see* inequality
power structures 132, 133
prejudice 23
primary care trust 129
primate studies 126–128, 131
primitive defence mechanisms 74–75
private medicine 161–162
production systems 179
productivity, and kindness 45
professional kindness 185–187
projection of feelings 56
projective identification 76–78
promoting
  kindness 157
  kinship 112–113
pseudo teams 79
psychiatric institutions 105–106
psychological defence mechanisms
    see defence mechanisms
psychosis *see* mental illness
psychosocial enterprises 179
psychotherapy, IAPT example 158–161
punishment 70–71, 100
purchase–provider split 148
pure systems approach 167
Putnam, Robert 23–24

Quality Improvement Network of
    Therapeutic Communities 168–170
quality-adjusted life years (QALYs) 144
quantitative/qualitative research 42–43
quotations
  Anonymous 100
  Bertrand Russell 82
  Department of Health 18
  Friedrich Nietzsche 68
  Lou Holtz 33
  Milan Kundera 51
  Phillips and Taylor 154
  Raymond Chandler 33
  Raymond Tallis 115
  Tony Blair 125
  William Shakespeare 9, 56, 139

rationalisation of behaviour 56
reaction formation 56
recession 16, 28
reciprocity 13, 16
reflective practice groups 80
reform, healthcare 1, 29, 187, 188
refugees 101–102
regulation 142, 162
  and autonomy 170–171
  balanced approaches 172–174, 178, 180
  dangers 165

regulating 177–179
  self 168
  simplified 189
  and trust 164
  see also freedom to serve
Reith Lectures, BBC 142, 144–145, 162–163
relationships
  to authority 70–71
  internal working models 41
  nurse–patient 130
  team boundaries 86
  see also therapeutic alliance
religion 11, 16
reparation 52, 59
repression 56, 72, 75
resuscitation 116–117
resilience, team 78–79
resonance, with patient traits 60
respect for patients 36, 38
responsibility 1, 3
  and change 132, 136, 137
  nursing staff 130
  organisational changes for good 188
  and person-centred care 97
  and teamwork 62
rhetoric 132, 133
Ricoeur, Paul 187
risk
  aversion 22, 97, 107–108, 186
  shared 1, 26, 27
rituals, nursing 130, 131
role/s
  expectations 71–72
  modelling 64–65
Royal College of Paediatrics and Child
    Health 94
Royal College of Psychiatrists 106, 168–170
rules 167
Russell, Bertrand 82
Russia 19

Sandel, Michael 142, 143, 144–145, 148
scandals, medical 141
scapegoating 77, 105–106, 133, 135
schizophrenia *see* mental illness
Schwartz, Barry 21, 155–156, 167
Schwarz Center rounds 81
Second World War 15, 19, 139
secure attachment 41
Seddon, John 167
Seldon, Anthony 162
self
  awareness 82, 172
  blame 58–59
  compassion 62
  confidence 14
  interest 12
  overcoming 54, 100
  regulation 168
self-assigned impossible tasks 59

self-harming patients 60
The Selfish Gene (Dawkins) 13
senior citizens *see* elderly care
sentimentality 5, 16
sexual relationships, clinician–patient 60–61
shadow side 52–53
    see also unconscious motivations
Shakespeare, William 9, 56, 139
shared risk 1, 26, 27
Shipman, Harold 16, 139–140
silencing 183
skimping 150
Smile or Die (Ehrenreich) 41–42
social
    capital 23–25
    defence mechanisms *see* defence mechanisms
    division 22–23
    functioning, agonic/hedonic/
        agonistic 126–128, 131, 134, 137, 150
    mobility 23, 26
    network analysis 24–25
    pressure 69–70
    relationships *see* relationships
    tension, primate studies 126, 127
    see also teamwork
solidarity 136, 189
spending cuts 16, 28
The Spirit Level (Wilkinson and Pickett) 20, 30
splitting 76–78, 107–110, 112, 119
stability, and change, system 134, 135
staff turnover 132, 133
standardisation
    competitive regulation dangers 165, 167, 172
    of tools 159
standards
    collaborative 169–170
    simplified 189
statistics, use/presentation 30
status 21, 22, 96–97
Sticks and Stones documentary 104
stigma 101, 105, 108, 112
Stoke Mandeville Hospital 133
stress 44–45
    chronic 21–22
    defence mechanisms 75
    and efficiency 181
    and kindness 43
    staff support groups 81
    supervision/support 66
    training/education 65
structural change *see* change, system
structural integration 90–91
subdivision of labour 159–160
sublimation, feelings 56
supervision, healthcare professionals 65–66
support, healthcare professionals 65–66
    groups 80–81
survival of the fittest 13–14
suspicion, culture of 23, 162–163
    see also trust/mistrust
system/s

fragmented 84–85, 87, 118, 149, 167
overload 132–134
    see also change; cooperation/fragmentation
Systems Thinking in the Public Sector (Seddon) 167

taboo of death 115, 121
Tallis, Raymond 54, 115, 116
target-setting 155, 186
Taylor, Barbara 12, 14
teamwork 10, 66, 82, 171
    boundaries 85–86, 87
    defence mechanisms 74–75
    denial 74, 75–76
    dynamics 68–69, 74, 81, 82
    fragmented systems 84–85
    group pressures 69–70
    healthy 79–80, *80*
    hunter-gatherer heritage 72–73
    and kindness 43
    leadership 97–98
    narrowing down primary task 86–87
    projective identification/splitting 76–78
    relationships to authority 70–71
    resilience 78–79
    role expectations 71–72
    shared responsibility of 62
    supervision 66
    support groups 80–81
    unconscious motivations 69, 73–74, 74–75
techno-centrism 161
technology of kindness 4
tension, social, primate studies 126, 127
therapeutic alliance 3, 44, *45*
    dependency/loneliness in patients 60–61
    and kindness 38–40, 43, *44*, *45*
    and placebo effect 42
    see also nurse–patient relationships
therapeutic environment 79, *80*
thinking/thought
    polarisation 101
    positive 41–42, 136
    see also unconscious motivations
threat-focus, hunter-gatherer heritage 72
    see also fear/uncertainty
time shortages/pressures 111, 160
token gestures 81–82
top-down change 128, 129–130, 133
Tormented Lives documentary 104
torture victims 101–102, 103
toxic environments 14, 178, 185, 186
training/education 62–65, 80–81
tribalism 73
trust/mistrust 23, *45*, 109
    and anxiety 43, 44
    crisis of 162–163
    and leadership 183
    patient 38, 39–40
    see also fear/uncertainty
Trust: How We Lost It And How To Get It Back (Seldon) 162

tunnel vision 166
turning a blind eye 140–141
  see also denial
turnover, staff 132, 133

UK Office for Budget Responsibility 28
The Unbearable Lightness of Being (Kundera) 51
uncertainty *see* fear/uncertainty
unconditional
  love 62
  positive regard 39, 42
unconscious motivations 52–53
  change 131
  defence mechanisms 56–57, 118
  over-identification 57–58
  projective identification/splitting 77
  scapegoating 105
  teamwork 69, 73–74, 74–75
undeserving patients 60, 100
unintended consequences 166–168
USA 19, 24, 29–30, 80–81

values 1, 139
vicious circles 109
Victorian period 12
virtues 11
virtuous circles 43–46, *44, 45*
  cooperation and fragmentation 90
  primate studies 126
  regulating regulation 179
  staff support groups 81
  and workplace culture 125

vocation 52
  commodification of 146–148
  and motivation 52–55

waiting times 165, 166
war
  metaphor 10
  Second World 15, 19, 139
Ward Atmosphere Scale 79
'Wards of the roses' 36
websites
  Abu Ghraib prison 72
  Agenda for Change 146
  group analytic approach 82
  Liverpool Care Pathway 120
  patient satisfaction 34
  Schwartz 156
welfare state 139
  see also National Health Service
whole-system perspectives 92
wilderness metaphor 105–106
Wilkinson, Richard 20, 30
Winnicott, Donald 61–62
workplace culture 125
wounded healers 52–53, 59

Yarl's Wood Immigration Removal
  Centre 103–104
yes we can slogan 29

zero tolerance 59
Zimbardo, Philip 71